D0889741

earch and Training Clinic

THE SELF IN PROCESS

THE SELF IN PROCESS

Toward a Post-Rationalist Cognitive Therapy

VITTORIO F. GUIDANO

THE GUILFORD PRESS
New York   London

© 1991 The Guilford Press
A Division of Guilford Publications, Inc.
72 Spring Street, New York, NY 10012

Printed in the United States of America

This book is printed on acid-free paper.

Last digit is print number: 9 8 7 6 5 4 3 2 1

Library of Congress Cataloging-in-Publication Data

Guidano, V. F.
    The self in process: toward a post-rationalist cognitive therapy
/ Vittorio F. Guidano.
        p.   cm.
    Includes bibliographical references and index.
    ISBN 0-89862-447-9
    1. Cognitive therapy.   2. Self psychology.   I. Title.
    [DNLM: 1. Cognitive Therapy.   2. Self Concept.   WM 425 G946s]
RC489.C63G85   1991
616.89'142—dc20
DNLM/DLC
for Library of Congress   90-14129
                                                              CIP

Preface

Although the powerful development of the cognitive sciences that has taken place over the last two decades has succeeded in fostering more articulated models of human behavior and knowing processes, the nature of human experience and the role that affectivity, meaning, and so forth, play in its construction are domains that have remained largely overlooked.

What the nature and structure of human experience might be is, in fact, a question that is not even asked in the empiricist epistemological perspective underlying the prevailing rationalist trend in cognitive psychology. If reality is taken as a univocal, objectively given, external order that exists independently from our observation of it, we will inevitably take for granted our own characteristics as observers. The only possible kind of investigation remaining in the face of something "already objectively given" is that of limiting oneself to the observation of various aspects of that given; and the most likely methodology resulting from this is that in which the description ends up coinciding with the explanation. Thus, describing the intercurrent mechanism between environmental stimuli and their sensory registration substantially amounts to the same as explaining the human sensory system. In the same way, describing human identity as merely an organized set of cognitions, perceptions, and memories correlated to a correspondent repertoire of feelings, emotional experiences, and psychophysiological patterns amounts to the same as explaining the nature and structure of selfhood.

If, on the other hand, we assume a nonempiricist perspective, the essential point becomes instead that of understanding how our characteristics as observers are involved in the process of observing, and this brings us to a radical change in the formulation followed up to now. It is not so much a question of describing what we feel or the ingredients that appear in individual identity, but rather one of asking why we feel what we feel, or why it is necessary to have a unitary sense of self continuous in time in order to be able to function. In other words, the unavoidable question becomes: "What is human experience?", and the only possible answer lies in researching the underlying mechanisms and processes causative of the phenomena (i.e., human experience) to be explained.

Hence, the assumption of an evolutionary epistemological perspective—that is, the study of evolving knowledge and knowing systems—necessarily becomes the basic methodological stance, given that, emphasizing how we cannot escape our particular way of being animal, such a stance enables the reconstruction of the human embeddedness of human experience. Moreover, if the ordering of our world is inseparable from our experiencing it, then the development of knowledge unfolds into an irreducible ontological dimension in which subjectivity underlies any ordering of that objective dimension of reality commonly called human experience.

This interdependence between subjective and objective, emotioning and cognizing, experiencing and explaining, etc., is constitutive of any human knowing process, just as feeling ourselves to be alive and the continuous explanation of this is constitutive of our nature and is at the base of our experience of selfhood. Because understanding is inseparable from existing, all understanding is self-understanding. The experiencing/explaining interdependence underlying self-understanding unfolds into an endless process of circularity between the immediate experience of oneself (the acting and experiencing "I") and the sense of self that emerges as a result of appraising and self-referring that ongoing experience (the observing and evaluating "Me").

This crucial feature inherent in selfhood dynamics is the essential thread around which the two parts of this book revolve. In Part I, which is of a theoretical nature, we attempt to outline the dynamics of the experiencing/explaining interface in selfhood development as well as the role that affectivity, meaning, and so forth, exert on the whole process. In Part II, of a more clinical nature, we try to show how working in a therapeutic setting on the experiencing/explaining interface may be a promising alternative to the rationalist methodics, essentially "persuasive" in nature, still largely adopted in cognitive therapy.

In conclusion, this book attempts to point out some of the basic features and essential processes that underlie human experience with a twofold intent: firstly, that of presenting an ontological model of knowledge in which knowing is seen from the point of view of the experiencing subject (i.e., how an individual experiences and is affected by the self-knowledge he or she has been able to process); secondly, that of deriving, in a manner consistent with the model presented, a methodology and strategy of intervention for cognitive therapy.

I wish to express my gratitude to the Center for Cognitive Therapy of Rome for the support and collaboration given me, and, in particular, to Giampiero Arciero, who, with involvement equal to enthusiasm, has sustained me throughout the drafting of this book with continual advice and suggestions.

There are many colleagues and friends to whom I owe thanks, and it would be impossible to name them all. I recall with particular gratitude the help of John Bowlby, Walter B. Weimer, Antonio Caridi, Toto Blanco, Jeremy Safran, Mayte Miró Barrachina, Oscar F. Goncalves, Mauro Ceruti, and Valeria Ugazio.

I extend special thanks to Michael J. Mahoney, both to celebrate a decade of friendship and to emphasize how this friendship has profoundly influenced my personal and scientific development.

I should also like to thank all my trainees, with whom I have discussed at length, and always profitably, the main ideas contained in this book.

There are many people to whom I am grateful for having made the editing and publishing work stimulating. Particular thanks to Matthew Dallaway for helping me put the work into the final English form; the readiness and professional competence of the staff of The Guilford Press, together with the unconditional support and friendship of Seymour Weingarten, have considerably eased the whole operation.

V. F. G.

essentially "persuasive" in nature, still largely adopted in cognitive therapy.

In conclusion, this book attempts to point out some of the basic features and essential processes that underlie human experience with a twofold intent: firstly, that of presenting an ontological model of knowledge in which knowing is seen from the point of view of the experiencing subject (i.e., how an individual experiences and is affected by the self-knowledge he or she has been able to process); secondly, that of deriving, in a manner consistent with the model presented, a methodology and strategy of intervention for cognitive therapy.

I wish to express my gratitude to the Center for Cognitive Therapy of Rome for the support and collaboration given me, and, in particular, to Giampiero Arciero, who, with involvement equal to enthusiasm, has sustained me throughout the drafting of this book with continual advice and suggestions.

There are many colleagues and friends to whom I owe thanks, and it would be impossible to name them all. I recall with particular gratitude the help of John Bowlby, Walter B. Weimer, Antonio Caridi, Toto Blanco, Jeremy Safran, Mayte Miró Barrachina, Oscar F. Goncalves, Mauro Ceruti, and Valeria Ugazio.

I extend special thanks to Michael J. Mahoney, both to celebrate a decade of friendship and to emphasize how this friendship has profoundly influenced my personal and scientific development.

I should also like to thank all my trainees, with whom I have discussed at length, and always profitably, the main ideas contained in this book.

There are many people to whom I am grateful for having made the editing and publishing work stimulating. Particular thanks to Matthew Dallaway for helping me put the work into the final English form; the readiness and professional competence of the staff of The Guilford Press, together with the unconditional support and friendship of Seymour Weingarten, have considerably eased the whole operation.

V. F. G.

Contents

II. PSYCHOTHERAPEUTIC PRINCIPLES

I

THEORETICAL PREMISES

. . . we are not like a tree which lives but does not feel, for whom earth, sun, air, rain and wind do not seem to be anything that they are not, that is, either friendly or else harmful things. We men instead are born to a sorry privilege, that of feeling ourselves to be alive, with the resultant great illusion: that is, to take as an external reality what is in fact an internal feeling of ours for life, and is changeable and varied, according to the times, our situation and our luck.

—L. PIRANDELLO, *The Late Mattia Pascal* (1904/1987, p. 159)

I

THEORETICAL PREMISES

. . . we are not like a tree which lives but does not feel, for whom earth, sun, air, rain and wind do not seem to be anything that they are not, that is, either friendly or else harmful things. We men instead are born to a sorry privilege, that of feeling ourselves to be alive, with the resultant great illusion: that is, to take as an external reality what is in fact an internal feeling of ours for life, and is changeable and varied, according to the times, our situation and our luck.

—L. PIRANDELLO, *The Late Mattia Pascal* (1904/1987, p. 159)

1

Selfhood Processes: An Ontological Approach

PRELIMINARY REMARKS

Cognitive psychology is, for the most part, still firmly anchored in the empiricist tradition and its basic postulates: (1) that an unequivocally given external reality exists in which a "sense of things" is objectively contained; and (2) that this reality can be observed from outside and assimilated, resulting in a univocal, objective understanding.

The information-processing perspective endorsed by proponents of the dominant rationalistic/computational approach represents the most current development based on these assumptions. This approach decrees that reality consists of a mind-independent ordered set of objects, knowledge about which coincides with a parallel set of internal representations derived from the progressive processing of external information. The validity (or truth) of knowledge as defined by its degree of correspondence to external reality inevitably leads to the positing of an outside, impartial viewpoint, making it possible to analyze individual knowledge independently of the individual possessing it (the so-called "God's eye point of view"; Putnam 1981). This emphasis on the correspondence principle necessarily implies primacy of the environment, on the basis of which adaptation becomes an externally regulated process, consisting of the continuous modeling of a knowing system to environmental pressures.

However, the interdisciplinary convergence that has taken place in recent years has resulted in some remarkable epistemological changes in the concepts of "reality" and "observer." These changes have rendered untenable a theory of the validity of knowledge that excludes the influence of the knowing subject (Hayek, 1952; Gadamer, 1979; Jantsch, 1980; Maturana, 1988a; Maturana & Varela, 1987; Weimer, 1979).

Reality is no longer thought of as unequivocal and ultimately objective, but as a network of interwoven multidirectional processes, simultaneously articulated along multiple levels of interaction. As Maturana (1986) makes clear, the radical shift is from an independent *universum* to a co-evolving *multiversa*, in which each versum is equally valid and unique. In other words, we live in a plurality of possible worlds and personal realities created by our own perceived distinctions. There are as many domains of existence as there are types of distinction constructed by the observer.

Consequently, the observer can no longer be assigned the privileged position of one who watches from the outside; indeed, any observing introduces into the network of interwoven processes an ordering distinction through which all of the possible ambiguities caused by the multiple, simultaneous interactions acquire, to the observer's eyes, an unequivocal and necessary character. Any observation—far from being "external" and therefore "objective"—is *self-referential.* It always reflects itself, that is, the perceiving order on which it is based, rather than the intrinsic qualities of the perceived object. Consequently, the order and regularity with which we habitually deal with things, as well as with ourselves, are not external and objectively given, but are rather a product of our continuous interaction with ourselves and the world. Thus, the historical relativity of knowing processes depends exclusively on their interactive and constructive nature, as is clearly expressed by the well-known aphorism of the Chilean School: "Everything said is said by an observer to another observer, who also could be him/herself" (Maturana, 1978, p. 31).

ONTOLOGY OF OBSERVING AND THE STRUCTURE OF HUMAN EXPERIENCE

Given that we can perceive the reality in which we live only from within our perceiving order, human experience arises from the *praxis* of our living which, in this sense, represents the absolutely inescapable primary ontological condition:

> We find ourselves as human beings here and now in the praxis of living, in language languaging, in *a priori* experiential situations in which everything that is, everything that happens, is and happens in us as part of our praxis of living. In these circumstances, whatever we say about how anything happens takes place in the praxis of our living as a comment, as a reflection, as a reformulation; in short, as an explanation of the praxis of our living, and as such it does not replace or constitute the praxis of living that it purports to explain. (Maturana, 1986, pp. 3–4)

Human beings cannot separate themselves from the way they view life, both because of their previous experience as a result of their praxis of living, and because they are part of a specific historical tradition. Hence, any understanding is always the result of interpretation: neither "subjective" (particular to the individual) nor "objective" (independent of the individual) (Winograd & Flores, 1986). Such an interpretation is the emerging product of the process of mutual regulation continuously alternating between *experiencing* and *explaining*, through which ongoing patterns of activity (immediate experiencing) become subject to distinctions and references, bringing about a reordering (explanation) which is able to change the very experiencing of the patterns themselves. As Maturana (1986) emphasizes, at the level of immediate experiencing it is not possible to distinguish between perception and illusion. Thus, for example, the perturbing feeling of having fleetingly seen a ghost is, for the subject who *is feeling* it, an irrefutable experience; only by shifting to the meta-experiential level of intersubjective coordination of thoughts and actions through languaging, can the individual explain the experience in terms of, let us say, a trick of the light, thus managing to transform and assimilate it into the perceived continuity of his or her praxis of living. In other words, understanding is not separable from human experience, so that to exist means literally to know. Hence, rather than representing a "given" reality according to a logic of external correspondence, knowing is the continous construction and reconstruction of a reality capable of making consistent the ongoing experience of the ordering individual (Arciero, 1989; Arciero & Mahoney, 1989; Mahoney, Miller, & Arciero, in press; Winograd & Flores, 1986; Varela, 1987).

Even though they both belong to our praxis of living, experiencing and explaining are, however, appraised in different ways by each person; explaining, entailing conscious distinctions, is self-referred as one's own internal activity, while experiencing, being so intertwined with our ordering of the world, is usually "outer-referred" to a single, external reality common to everybody.

> Consider, for example, a group of people attending a symphonic concert. The experiences of the various people will vary depending on their interests, backgrounds, current state, etc. Some of the things they experience will pertain to the sights of the hall and the members of the orchestra, the sounds and beauty of the music, and the total atmosphere of the concert hall. Whatever experience each person has phenomenologically, the colors, sounds, beauty and atmosphere will appear to them to be occurring outside of themselves (that is, in terms of naive realism). But everything just mentioned occurs solely within the conscious experiences produced by the nervous systems of the people in the hall. . . . The human reality of the concert, in other words, is a construction of the brain. It is both created by and experienced in the brain . . . our nervous system is responsible for constructing the reality of the human environment. (Ritter, 1979, pp. 203–204)

Hence, moment-by-moment understanding unfolds through a circular process in which an immediate and tacit perception of self and world (*a priori* first-order experiences) through explicit linguistic abilities is reordered and scaffolded in terms of propositions distributed within conceptual networks; this reordering makes possible new dimensions of experience, such as "true–false," "subjective–objective," etc. (*a posteriori* second-order experiences).

In all living beings, the affective-emotional system corresponds to an immediate and irrefutable perception of the world. Therefore, from an ontological point of view, feelings can never be mistaken, since through them we can directly experience our way of being, so that we always are as we feel we are (Olafson, 1988, p. 109). Errors can be noticed only *a posteriori*, and depend on the point of view that we, as observers, take in reordering our experiencing. Hence any rational-cognitive reordering (explaining) consists of operating with the coherence of semanticological rules based on premises tacitly provided by immediate experiencing and accepted *a priori*. Every rational system therefore has an emotional base, and this explains why nobody can be convinced by a logical argument if they have not already accepted its premise *a priori* (Maturana, 1988b).

Conscious-explicit restructuring makes new levels of abstraction available, transforming the continuous modulation of internal states into patterns of self-understanding that modify ongoing immediate experience and facilitate its further articulation. Thus, while experiencing would appear to be a necessary constraint for any explanation, explaining is in turn crucial in giving consistency and meaning to life events. As Dostoevski noted over a century ago in *Memories from Underground*, no one can do without explaining to themselves what is happening to them, and if one day they should no longer be able to explain anything to themselves, they would say they had gone mad, and this would be for them the last explanation left.

Hence, experiencing and explaining, although different in terms of "embedded immediacy" versus "abstracted distancing," are polarities which are ever present in the endless circularity of our understanding, whether we are dealing with externals or with ourselves. Now, the experience of "being-a-self" is something intertwined with and arising from our praxis of living, so that, as Gadamer (1976) says, "the self that we are does not possess itself: one could say that it *happens*" (p. 55).

The experiencing/explaining interdependence underlying self-understanding is matched by an endless process of circularity between the immediate experience of oneself (the acting and experiencing "I") and the sense of self that emerges as a result of abstractly self-referring the ongoing experience (the observing and evaluating "Me") (James, 1890; Mead, 1934; Smith, 1978, 1985). The self as subject ("I") and as object ("Me") therefore emerge as irreducible dimensions of a selfhood dynamic whose directionality depends on the ongoingness of our praxis of living. Indeed, the acting and experiencing "I" is always one step ahead of the current appraisal of the situation, and the evaluating "Me" becomes a continuous process or reordering and reconstructing one's conscious sense of self.

We will now go on to outline briefly the theoretical framework that can be developed out of the ontological perspective advanced above.

AN EVOLUTIONARY APPROACH
TO SELFHOOD PROCESSES

The epistemological change in the observer–observed relationship, highlighting the co-dependence of knowledge and order from the very beginning, has brought a new branch of epistemology to the fore: evolutionary epistemology (see Campbell, 1974). This is an approach that uses and relates data from cognitive, biological, and evolutionary science to trace patterns and processes underlying the interdependence of evolving knowledge and knowing systems, so that such a methodology is also defined by the terms "natural" (Maturana, 1978) or "experimental" epistemology (Ceruti, 1989; Radnitzky & Bartley, 1987). In effect, the application of an evolutionary perspective in order to understand the nature of knowing and the manner of its acquisition reveals that knowledge itself has evolved along with other aspects of life, and is now recognized as a specific field of the natural sciences (Lorentz, 1973; Piaget, 1971; Popper, 1972, 1975, 1982; Popper & Eccles, 1977). Quite rightly, therefore, Weimer (1982) has suggested that epistemology has every right to be considered one of the psychological sciences, and, in particular, that evolutionary epistemology should form the basis for any consistent methodology of cognitive psychology.

The fact that any knowing reflects the specific self-referent constraints through which a living system scaffolds its own reality, allows us to put the problem of selfhood emergence in biological terms as well as in terms of psychological processes, definitively removing any "metaphysical" or "intuitionist" implications which for a long time precluded its study. Indeed, if knowing is distributed along a continuum ranging from early rudimentary exploratory behavior to human self-consciousness, then evolution emerges as an essential regulatory strategy aimed at achieving stability in an ever-changing medium through the attainment of more complex levels of autonomous self-referent functioning.

> Selfhood is a necessary consequence of structurally complex systems that satisfy certain constraints. That we know selves as embodied by the highest primates is, in effect, due to local factors in this region of the universe; selves could be embodied quite differently. (Weimer, 1982, p. 352)

The crucial point for understanding selfhood dynamics "in this region of the universe" lies in the notion of *self-organization*, according to which living systems, as a result of a basic evolutionary constraint, organize themselves and work to preserve their systemic identity/integrity (Atlan, 1979, 1981, 1984; Jantsch, 1980; Nicolis & Prigogine, 1977; Maturana & Varela, 1980; Varela, 1979).

Plainly, the temporal becoming of any individual knowing system should be regarded as the unfolding of a self-organizing process that, through the maturational development of higher cognitive abilities, progressively constructs a sense of self-identity endowed with inherent unique features and historical continuity, whose maintenance becomes as important as life itself. The interdependence of selfhood and knowledge processes makes it possible for the generation and assimilation of information to be regulated by self-identity patterns thus far structured, and this in turn makes possible the continuous ordering of experience along a unitary and coherent dimension.

On the other hand, self-organizing in terms of internal coherence implies that all the possible pressures for change that emerge as a consequence of the ongoing assimilation of experience are subordinate to the maintenance of the "experiential order" (personal meaning) on which rests the perceived consistency and continuity of one's self. Thus, a self-organizing system can reach an interactional equilibrium in an ever-changing reality to the extent to which environmental pressures trigger viable changes in its experiential order that facilitates the emergence of more integrated levels of self-identity and self-consciousness.

Adaptation, therefore, is the ability to transform perturbation arising from interaction with the world into information meaningful to one's experiential order. Maintaining an adaptive adequacy essentially means preserving one's sense of self by continuously transforming the perceived world rather than merely corresponding to it. This explains why the notion of the *viability* of knowing processes has become much more important in recent evolutionary epistemology than that of their *validity* (see Zeleny, 1981).

Finally, the lifespan development of a human system is regulated by an orthogenetic progression (Brent, 1978, 1984; Prigogine, 1976; Werner, 1948, 1957); that is, shifts in experience assimilation produced by systemic reorganizations of ongoing patterns of internal coherence eventually result in the discontinuous emergence of more inclusive levels of the knowledge of self and of the world. The development of this progression in many ways resembles the pattern of "punctuated equilibria" proposed by post-Darwinian pluralistic evolutionary approaches (see Gould, 1980). In actual fact, lifespan development does not reflect a smooth curve of cumulative acquisition of knowledge so much as a discontinuous curve in which periods of relative structural stability are "punctuated" by episodes of whole-system upheaval in which major reorganizations (personal revolutions) emerge to become the next "tacit base-camp" of viability (Mahoney, 1991).

We will now briefly outline the essential aspects that underlie human self-organization of knowledge, that is, the "medium" in which selfhood takes on form, and the existential dimension through which it unfolds.

Intersubjectivity and Self-Individuation

In all primates a highly complex social world has been superimposed on the mere physical environment, bringing about an intersubjective reality in which knowing oneself and the world is always in relation to others. Thus the greater viability in ordering experience offered by synchronization and mutual coordination of actions is matched by an increase in intersubjective learning (imitation, modeling, etc.) as well as by an increase in the capacity for self-individuation. These capabilities became more and more indispensable as adaptation transformed itself into a social affair (Buss, 1987, 1988; Kummer, 1979; Passingham, 1982).

The ability to discriminate between individual others is hard-wired in the primate organization, as is clearly shown by evidence of the central role of the face in the primate emotional system. The progressive elaboration of neocortical mechanisms underlying the evolution of primate cognition does not depend on the replacement of innate behavior by learned behavior, but on the selection and control of innate behavior by conceptually stored information (Reynolds, 1981). Hence, facial recognition is a neocortical processing feature whose evolutionary progression closely parallels the emergence of more complex intersubjective dimensions (e.g., closer mother–infant relationships, competition and social bonds) which require a greater and greater capacity for attunement with others' behavior and intentions in order to reach a proper adaptation (e.g., attainment of secure attachments, adequate social ranks).

Facial recognition should therefore be regarded as a self-referent ordering of intersubjective experience that facilitates the possibility of self-individuation. On the one hand, the ability to discriminate between individual others allows one to anticipate their perception of one's actions, thus improving interactional synchrony and reciprocity. On the other hand, simulating how others will regard one's actions entails the capacity to view oneself from the perceived perspective of others. This enhances the possibilities for self-bordering and self-individuation.

Thus, in the co-evolution of intersubjectivity and individuation which are the distinguishing marks of primate organization, the ability to differentiate between self and others emerges as the essential condition for structuring a stable self-recognition. Studies in self-recognition processes using mirror-image techniques have shown that prior exposure to interaction with others is the fundamental requisite for great apes, placed in front of a mirror, to be able to refer the reflected image to themselves, thereby achieving a rudimentary, stable, self-individuation (Gallup, 1970, 1977; Gallup, McClure, Hill, & Bundy, 1971; Gallup & Suarez, 1986). Hence, in the continuum of primate evolutionary progression, facial recognition and mimicking are first steps in the mirror-image mechanism which, along with the emergence of language, gives rise to the more structured and integrated levels of self-recognition that characterize human self-awareness. One of the first clear manifestations of self-recognition in chimpanzees was seen in an experimental situation which required simultaneously a mirror-image (a capacity for self-referring) and a language (a capacity to operate distinctions in immediate experience) (Gardner & Gardner, 1971). Initially, the researchers had taught their young female chimp, Washoe, a sign language similar to the manual alphabet used for communication by deaf-mutes, which contained a number of words, including the name Washoe. Later she was put in front of a mirror, and to the question "Who's that?" Washoe replied, "It's Washoe," demonstrating ability both to distinguish the reflected image from immediate experience and to refer the former to the latter (Morin, 1986; Morin & Piatelli-Palmarini, 1974).

Basically, language is matched by the emergence of a new level of self-referent ordering according to lexical and semantic rules that allow for the restructuring of immediate experience in terms of propositions, that is, "objects" abstracted from space and time for which the predication of "truth" or "falsehood" is meaningful. The possibility of sharing common criteria for "truth" disengaged from the immediacy of experience makes possible, in its turn, the emergence of new dimensions in the reciprocal coordination of actions and intentions, as well as in the negotiation of mutual agreements.

> The basic function of language as a system of orienting behavior is not the transmission of information or the description of an independent universe about which we can talk, but the creation of a consensual domain of behavior between linguistically interacting systems through the development of a cooperative domain of interactions. (Maturana, 1978, p. 50)

Naturally, the dimension of intersubjective experience offered by language further articulates the already existing capacities for individuation and self-recognition, bringing about the development of a sense of self, both as a subject ("I") and as an object ("Me").

The increased ability for synchronic attunement with others' intentions through linguistic interactions is paralleled by an increased ordering of the flow of internal states and psychophysiological rhythms that lend continuity to immediate experiencing ("I"). Along with this, the capacity to view oneself from the perspectives of others is increased by linguistic abstracting abilities, giving rise to a recognizable sense of one's perceived continuity and sameness ("Me"). This capacity, disengaged from the immediacy of the interactional context, becomes an essential instrument for reordering immediate experience and stabilizing internal coherence.

In other words, self-consciousness should be regarded as an ontological process in which the ability to balance a distinction between immediate experience and its appraisal through interactions with others is matched by the ability to refer the experiencing "I" to the appraising "Me." Thus, while being an event of our praxis of living that is at once discursive and actional, self-consciousness is always consciousness of others, existing by means of language and within a historical context.

> The consciousness at work in decentered subjectivity is both linguistic and actional, embedded in a history of social practices. It thus borrows its being from the praxial history of speaking and acting subjects as they respond to the speech and action of others. Through this borrowing, consciousness is dialogically constituted. Admittedly, consciousness can be alone; it can fashion a soliloquy and it can monitor an individual act in solitude. In all this, consciousness is experienced as "mine." Yet, being alone is itself a peculiar modality of being with others; soliloquy is carried out by a language that belongs to the public, and individual acts have meaning only within the wider context of social practices. One can be alone only because one has already been

in communal interaction with others; one can speak "by" and "to" oneself only with a grammar that has a social history. (Schrag, 1986, p. 172)

Finally, the bipolarity of selfhood processes, in accordance with which the "I" comes to recognize itself as a "Me" through the "mirror-image" provided by others, makes an ontological, irreducible demarcation between "subjective" and "objective," "inner sense" and "outer sense," "experiencing" and "explaining" which is central to the unfolding of our praxis of living as human beings. A bipolar selfhood is found in both Eastern and Western conceptions of self; however, rather than attempting to differentiate it, the East tends to experience selfhood as simultaneously subjective and objective, while the West tends to differentiate the inside (self as subject) from the outside (self as object), consequently perceiving "external" objects as existing separately from the observer (Johnson, 1985).

Meaning as the Human Dimension of Existence

The most singular aspect of the human experience is its "effort after meaning," as is evident from both evolutionary and ontogenetic points of view.

As far as the evolutionary aspect is concerned, the emergence of language and reflexive self-referring—transforming the immediacy of living into an endless circularity between experiencing and explaining—makes the construction of meaning an essential ingredient of the process of self-individuation and self-recognition.

Human self-consciousness breaks the unity of people within Nature. Self-consciousness with forethought and afterthought gives rise to the human existential predicament. At least for the last 50,000 years, we and our forebears have faced the puzzle (which we have had the words to pose to ourselves) of whence we came into the world, why we are here and what happens when we die. But as we know, this is no matter of mere curiosity. Since reflective language made us persons, we have cared about ourselves and each other *as* persons. So, the inevitability of the eventual death of self and loved ones and the arbitrary unpredictability of death from famine, disease, accident, predation or human assault becomes the occasion not for momentary animal terror but for what is potentially unremitting human anguish. And the quest for meaning, for meanings compatible with a human life of self-conscious mortality, becomes a matter of life and death urgency. . . . Yet, contrary to the old myth, our forebears cannot have been cast out of Nature's Garden of Eden in a sudden, tragic "birth trauma." Even if the final full attainment of language competence worked itself out very rapidly once the basic structural-generative principles of human language had been hit upon, self-conscious selfhood, with its imperative challenge to find supportive meaning in the face of creature mortality, must have emerged over a period of time. If so, the symbolic resources of language-bearing human communities could meet the need for meaning as it arose. Thus emerged the many worlds of myth, ritual and religion that provided the traditional answers to the question of what it means to be human. (Smith, 1978b, p. 1055)

The social structure of human reality made it possible, right from the beginning, for the core meaning of being human to be founded on the emotions triggered by reciprocal interactions with others aimed at maintaining mutual coordination and consensus between people. The human quest for meaning should therefore be regarded as the development of a proactive understanding biased by a set of specific intersubjective constraints (parent–child relationships, social bonds, group cohesiveness, etc.) which define a range of prototypical emotions (attachment and love, bereavement and grief, etc.) for sharing meanings in terms of a shared symbolic-linguistic dimension.

At the individual level, this continuous search for meaning takes form in the lifespan construction and maintenance of a coherent personal meaning, that is to say, how the experiencing subject ("I") relates to the "meaning-of-being-human" as prescribed by the tradition in which it lives, able thereby to define and recognize itself in a continuous and unequivocal way ("Me"). Thus, on the one hand, the emotional modulation connected to the process of demarcation between self and others constrains the development of any personal dimension of meaning; on the other hand, the "I"/"Me" differentiation resulting from such demarcation corresponds to that type of ontological understanding included in the terms of personal meaning. Indeed, any differentiation of self-boundaries implies an ontological understanding (how the "Me" is able to appraise its experiencing "I") in which personal meaning represents the proactive process. That is, an ongoing ordering of networks of related meaningful events makes possible an experiencing of the world capable of triggering patterns of emotional modulation ("I") specifically recognizable as the unity and continuity in time of one's owns self ("Me").

In other words, from a self-organizing perspective, bringing forth a coherent world is the first and last condition for having a consistent self-identity, with personal meaning as the proactive understanding that reveals a specific mode of being becoming the key notion in the elaboration of an ontological theory of personality. This is what we shall try to do in the remaining chapters of the first part of this book.

2

The Differentiation of Self-Boundaries

Because the evolutionary and developmental human environment essentially corresponds to an interpersonal reality structured and made consistent by language, any knowledge of the world always rests on, and is mediated by, intersubjective experience. Any newborn human being would appear to be naturally endowed with the capacity for intersubjective experience, that is, with a hard-wired propensity for knowing people, and him- or herself in relation to others (Trevarthen, 1979, 1982). While self-knowledge has its epistemological foundation in the sense of similarity perceived in interaction with others (Cooley, 1902; Hamlyn, 1974; Mead, 1934), its ontological development takes place through an increasingly individualized process of differentiating one's own self from the common attributes and meanings shared with others—a unique differentiation from other ways of experiencing life (nonself) upon which rests the very possibility of self-perception. Becoming an ontological self corresponds to a self-referent ordering of the essential tension perceived in the interactional synchrony with others. Others' perceived similarity is the necessary requisite for experiencing a sense of personhood, but at the same time, the differentiation from such perceived similarity is the necessary condition for experiencing a sense of selfhood. The oscillative balance inherent in such self-referent ordering should be considered as an ongoing moment-to-moment result of the perpetual process of negotiating a mutual consensus with, and acceptance by, others. Throughout lifespan development, the self–nonself differentiation acts as the basic self-organizing principle that underlies the ontological process of psychological and existential individuation (self-identity and personal meaning).

In order to obtain a unified picture of the developmental dynamics of self-identity, it will be helpful to bear in mind the different—but closely interwoven—levels of the relevant processes:

1. The way in which structured interactions with specific others (attachment processes) are involved in the emergence of self, both as subject (the "I," i.e., the sense of self felt in an immediate and direct way) and as an object (the "Me," i.e., the self that one comes to know through one's own behavior).
2. The emotional and cognitive processes that articulate these subsystems into a specific self-referential process of personal meaning.

ATTACHMENT AND THE
DIFFERENTIATION OF SELF-BOUNDARIES

It now seems to be well established that, from the earliest phases of development, the infant is equipped with basic feelings, as well as the basic ability to communicate them through expressive-motor mechanisms that are mainly concentrated in the face system. The propensity for modulating environmental contingencies with feeling reactions expresses very well the infant's ability to become attuned with others, and in particular with significant others as caregivers (Buck, 1984; Ekman, 1972, 1984; Fox & Davidson, 1984; Izard, 1977, 1980; Reite & Field, 1985; Plutchik, 1984).

Effectively, the interdependency and reciprocity of psychophysiological rhythms between infant and caregiver appear to be inherently co-dependent and co-existing with the child's activity in ordering self and world perception from the very beginning (Bell & Ainsworth, 1972; Brazelton, Koslowski, & Main, 1974; Stayton, Hogan, & Ainsworth, 1971). Many data, moreover, indicate that even during gestation there is real "intrauterine learning" resulting from the fetus's active participation in such rhythmic reciprocity (Brazelton, 1983; Ianniruberto & Tajani, 1981; Milani Comparetti, 1981).

Considering knowledge as a self-organizing process (i.e., as a viable way of "bringing-forth-a-world" while "being-in-it") the strong tendency to make close emotional bonds with caregivers emerges as the fundamental ontological constraint that underlies any possible ordering of experience. Through the self-referent ordering carried out by his or her search for proximity to caregivers, the infant can border the dimensions of exchange with the world and perceive the sensory inflow along an approach–avoidance continuum centered and balanced on attachment figures. In other words, attuning oneself with an identifiable external source of cyclical rhythms transforms an otherwise unknowable space dimension into a highly personal reality made understandable by relatively simple physical parameters; thus, even the attribution of spatial qualities (proximity–distance) to the surrounding world rests on an intersubjective apperception of that world. At the same time, matching the flow of one's inner states against an ordered, external set of rhythms and intentions makes it possible to perceive recurrent regularities in that flow, and to modulate in more specific ways one's approach–avoidance oscillations. Again, any possible attribution of feeling qualities to ongoing psychophysiological reactions is matched by a perceived similarity to significant others.

Given that the search for proximity to caregivers and self-organizing abilities seem to be inextricably interwoven, it will be helpful to examine the intersubjective processes mediating the interdependency between attachment and selfhood.

Being equipped, as a primate, with neocortical processes that mediate facial recognition, the human infant from the moment of birth exhibits a specific ability to imitate caregivers' actions (Field et al., 1982). Rather than being an instinctive releasing mechanism (i.e., a passive coupling between a response and a specific stimulus display), neonate facial recognition and imitation are actually self-referent ordering activities. Through intermodal coordination, perceptual data from the visual system are connected with other perceptual modalities (e.g., proprioceptive feedback, psychophysiological modulation) and ordered into affective-motoric patterns of response (Meltzoff & Borton, 1979; Meltzoff & Moore, 1985; Zajonc & Markus, 1984). If facial recognition, as a behavioral pattern, already reflects a self-referent procedure for mapping and coordinating different sensorial modalities, it should be quite clear how, at a more organizational level, the reciprocal emotional attunement between caregivers' mimicking on the one hand and infant imitation on the other could be actively ordered, by the infant, into recurrent primordial units of self-perception.

The organizational role that attachment exerts, both in the

development of a sense of self as a subject ("I") and as an object ("Me"), can be outlined as follows:

While the attunement to a synchronous source of regularities organizes the sensory inflow into a stream of recurrent psychophysiological rhythms, the emotional aspects of attachment transform feeling tonalities into specific emotional modules. Through regularities drawn from caregivers' behavior and motivations, the infant can start to connect diffuse basic feelings to perceptions, actions and memories, turning them into specific emotional schemata susceptible to subjective experience. The emergence of subjective experience is matched by the perception that one is an entity differentiated from other objects and people in the surrounding world. Physiological rhythms and emotional schemata become basic ingredients of infantile consciousness, which is truly affective in nature and quality (Buck, 1984; Emde, 1984; Izard, 1980). The self-feeling immediately and directly perceived as an inner kinesthetic sense (the "I") is therefore primarily organized around prototypical emotional schemata differentiated out of the attachment reciprocity with caregivers.

The "I" comes to see him- or herself as a "Me" (i.e., like other surrounding persons) only through the consciousness that caregivers have of his or her behavior. Anticipating others' perception of one's actions facilitates the recognition of ongoing patterns of emotional schemata out of the stream of recurrent inner states, structuring them into specific emotional experiences connected to related intentions and goal-oriented behaviors. Evidence suggests that infants' perceptions of their image through caregivers' behavior are not confined to those situations in which parents attempt to meet their basic needs. Parents' imitation of infant behavior is very common from the earliest periods (Bretherton & Waters, 1985; Harter, 1983) and, very probably, such imitation is an essential cue allowing the infant to recognize as his or her own the characteristics and attitudes through which caregivers perceive him or her as a person. In other words, self-consciousness emerges from a self-recognizability made possible by the empathic ability to take the attitudes of others onto oneself; elaborating a conscious self-image consists of bordering the profile of the "Me" out of the perceived "I."

Self–other differentiation is a complex, multilevel process in which the actor's sense ("Me") of felt uniqueness and oneness ("I") is found both in attunement to others and in differentiation from others, both equally necessary conditions for its experiencing. On the one hand, the intersubjective process of knowing from understanding another person entails *identifying oneself with,* insofar as it always unfolds through empathic variables (feeling what another feels) supported and mediated by a perceived similarity with a significant other—that is, an emotional involvement with an attachment figure (Hoffman, 1975, 1978). On the other hand, perceiving the similarity of others' feelings as a requisite for recognizing the same feeling within the self means *bordering* one's subjectivity out of the objectivity of an interpersonal, sharable reality.

The notion of internal working models of attachment figures and self clearly implies the organization of a system for transforming intersubjective experience into personal knowledge (Bowlby, 1969, 1983, 1973, 1980; Bretherton & Waters, 1985). In this sense, an attachment figure does not correspond to an isomorphic representation within a specific sensorimotor modality of caregivers' behavior, as if it were a sort of perceptual entity mediating information about attachment-related events. On the contrary, internalizing an attachment figure within a rhythmic and self-regulating modulation of inner states actually involves shaping an intermodal patterning of sensory-motor-affective modules into a unified configuration that can result in a sense of self and the world.

Just as facial recognition is matched by a self-ordering in proprioception and body experience, similarly, imitating or identifying with another person corresponds to perceiving oneself as "being-in-the-world." A child, when appraising a stimulus situation by referencing the mother's face (*social referencing;* Campos & Stenberg, 1981; Klinnert et al., 1983), perceives a recognizable sense of his or her being in a specific situation through the understanding of the mother's affective state. Social referencing is therefore a basic process ordering the intersubjectivity inherent in the attachment system (i.e., the other's image corresponds to a perception of self).

Throughout development, any shifting of levels in intersubjective abilities (e.g., from the mere sense of others' existence to conceptual perspective-taking) is matched by a parallel increase in the capacity for empathic attunement (e.g., from imitation to identification). Feeling oneself emotionally involved in perceiving a similarity with significant others therefore seems to be the essential invariant underlying any development of ontological knowledge during the lifespan. In the concrete social referencing of maturational stages, the child's intersubjectivity is, to a large extent, bound to the immediate existential situation, so that the sense of being a unique and specific person is usually attained through an emotional identification with attachment figures. The abstract social referencing of adulthood, disengaging the individual from the current aspect of interaction, allows the attainment of a definite sense of personal reality through the construction of even more abstract perceived similarities to significant others, as in common love relationships. In any case, whether it be an emotional identification with another's image, or a more abstract construction, feeling oneself involved in a unique and exclusive interaction is crucial in bringing forth a sense of the world which is able to produce a quality of self-perception ("I") recognizable as one's own self ("Me"). In this sense, perceived uniqueness of significant bonds may function in a manner analogous to the syntactic principles of organization that underlie a semantic structure of understanding (Marris, 1982), thus exerting an essential role in the development of any affective relationship.

THE ORGANIZATIONAL UNITY OF THE EMOTIONAL DOMAIN

In a space–time dimension apprehensible in terms of proximity–distance from an attachment safe-base, the psychobiological attunement to caregivers allows the newborn human primate to order its sensory inflow into feelings decodable only on an approach–avoidance continuum. In primates, where any ordering of reality is matched by intersubjective experience, attachment acts by regulating the rhythmic oscillation between arousal-inducing (exploration, play) and arousal-reducing (security, clinging) psychophysiological patterns, as well as by modulating fear and anger by switching these same patterns (Fox & Davidson, 1984; Reynolds, 1981; Suomi, 1984).

At the human level, the structure and quality of early emotional reciprocity inherent in ongoing patterns of attachment is closely correlated to the infant's experience of caregivers' accessibility in response to his or her need for proximity and contact. Out of the great variety of possible responses by parents to that search for contact, constrained by the infant's limited scheme of reference, a finite set of experiences about caregivers' availability evolves. That is, the access to caregivers is felt as *secure* and so is the attachment exhibited; or the access is experienced as *blocked* and the infant exhibits an *insecure-avoidant* attachment; or the access is perceived as *unpredictable* and it is matched by an *insecure-ambivalent* attachment (Ainsworth et al., 1978; Bretherton, 1985; Main, Kaplan, & Cassidy, 1985). The presence of true central attachment organizations from the earliest stages of development clearly demonstrates the self-regulatory and self-organizing capabilities exhibited by attachment processes. Essentially, these consist of assembling various patterns of arousal-inducing and arousal-reducing modules, adjusting their modulation through anger and fear (i.e., ambivalent or avoidant attachments) to produce a viable level of emotional reciprocity (security proximity).

A central attachment organization is the emergent result of a process of selection and stabilization from the flow of recurrent internal states and psychophysiological rhythms of patterns of self-perception, making them available to appraisal and recognition by the experiencing subject. In other words, if an attachment relationship is a self-referential process for "having-a-world" while "being-in-it," then the stability of attachment patterns exhibited by an infant reflects a way of "bringing-forth-a-world" capable of producing a quality of self-perception ("I") recognizable as one's own self ("Me").

Bordering the "Me" while organizing the "I" is a complex and multilevel developmental process that gradually unfolds as the infant achieves self-recognition (e.g., the ability to recognize and respond to the self independently from the immediate perceptual contingencies; Bertenthal & Fischer, 1978; Lewis & Brooks-Gunn, 1979). The emerging ability to perceive oneself within a feeling of permanence and continuity in space–time (cf. the Piagetian stage of object permanence) is matched by an increased awareness of the differentiation between self and others, as reflected by the first surfacing of the fear of strangers, preeminently the "others" (Wolf, 1982). An increased awareness of others as distinct objects is matched by an increased understanding that one is a distinct object too.

A quite stable, even though rudimentary, sense of self allows the unfolding of a new level of self-referentiality, that of starting to refer to oneself the immediacy of one's experiencing ("I"), thus being able to begin recognizing it ("Me"). In other words, the felt sense of self, once it can be focused and appraised, can give rise to a second order of self-referred experiences: self-explanations, that is, a reorder of immediate experience which makes it recognizable and understandable. Thus, self-recognition is actually bordering from the perceived distinctness of others a definite sense of individuality ("Me") out of one's unique and pervasive feeling of being apart ("I").

If we consider human knowledge from an ontological perspective, we can affirm that in the human lifespan, self-recognition is the first explanation we manage to give ourselves of our feeling of being alive. We are thus dealing with a primary ontological differentiation in which a fairly stable sense of self-recognition results from an equally stable demarcation between self-perception (the "inner sense" subjectively felt) and world-perception (the "outer sense" objectively experienced with others). The integration of inner and outer senses, crucial in the maintenance of one's internal coherence, allows for an even more articulated self-referentiality in knowing processes. Thus, any information from world perception corresponds to information about the self (e.g., how others' perceptions regulate the appraisal of the "Me") and, conversely, a self-knowledge development parallels the process by which the individual comes to understand reality (e.g., how the organizational content of the "I" influences the structuring of defining features of self and world).

The stabilization of a sense of self, which parallels the process of self-recognition, takes place through the assembling of psychophysiological motor rhythms, and sensory, motor and emotional modules, into a self-ordering core of affective, autonomic, and behavioral activity. Clusters of emotional schemata (e.g., prototypical affect-laden scenes abstracted from events and situations repeatedly experienced) are ordered into an oscillative, recursive loop capable both of generating a sense of self-perception matched with specific emotions and behaviors, and of self-regulating through the rhythmic activation/deactivation of its opponent feeling tonalities (Mineka et al., 1981; Solomon, 1980). Thus, the avoidant attitude exhibited by children of rejecting parents is the dynamic moment-to-moment balancing between opponent emotional states, like attachment and anger, aimed at preserving the level of emotional reciprocity compatible with the inaccessibility perceived in the relationship. The rhythmic interplay between opponent emotional states is *internal* to the infant and has no direct reference to the present course of the relationship; it is as though the contact itself arouses anger and withdrawal, and withdrawal leads again to contact that leads again to anger and withdrawal (Cassidy & Kobak, 1988; Main & Weston, 1982). The ability to maintain and regulate one's sense of self rests on the organizational unity which the developing emotional domain acquires from the very beginning.

The rhythmic and oscillative interplay between basic ensembles of opponent emotional schemata provides the decoding context for the further differentiation of a whole set of discrete emotions. That is, emotional differentiation appears as a match-to-pattern process between preformed emotional schemata and ongoing feelings. The search for internal coherence, biasing any possible decoding pattern, acts as the main regulator, giving unity and functional continuity in time to the whole development, while the perception of discrepancy acts as the essential trigger for differentiating new emotional tonalities (Guidano, 1987). On the other hand, the decentralized control that governs the recursive loop of modular processing units allows the maintenance of a sense of self through a recombination of these modules within various subsytems. Thus, the activation of anger, although specifically constrained by a perceptual key as rejection or the threat of it, may become part of the patterns of attachment (Reynolds, 1981; Sander, 1975) as well as of exploration and play (Suomi, 1984), supplying continuity and unity to the immediate experience of oneself. In the process, the gradual unfolding of concrete cognitive abilities lends further stability to the current sense of self, and schooling and peer relationships, progressively broadening the experiential domains, foster the progressive articulation of that sense of self.

Once the sense of self that emerges through a central attachment organization has stabilized, a more structured and articulated level of self-referentiality regulates the dynamics between subjective and objective boundaries of the self, bringing about new dimensions of intersubjective experience, and hence of self-knowledge. Being able to differentiate between the subjectivity of the immediate experience of oneself and the objectivity of caregivers' perception of oneself entails the self-referent reordering of one's immediate experiencing ("I") as if it were an object ("Me"), that is, from the perceived viewpoint of caregivers. The psychophysiological and affective modulation provided by the rhythmic oscillation between prototypical emotional schemata may be appraised through a definite sense of self resulting from the increasing awareness of one's distinctness from others. In this way, a continuous reordering of one's immediate experience to make it consistent with that sense of self becomes possible. Any reordering of immediate experience takes place at the level of explicit knowledge procedures made available by gradual cognitive growth; that is, the experienced consequences of events and actions are abstracted into a conceptual cause–effect frame and stored in accessible, manipulable form (expectations, beliefs, procedures for problem solving, etc.). Explicit knowing procedures are self-referential processes aimed at making ongoing tacit experience consistent; that is, the processing of expectations, beliefs, etc., is the essential modality for trying to appraise and recognize the immediate experience of any given situation and to make it coherent with one's own sense of continuity.

Thus, as the developmental processes become more complex and multidirectional, more integrative conceptual devices become necessary to support an overall dynamic view, both of the interdependence between affect and cognition, and of the part it plays in the differentiation of self-boundaries. In our opinion, if viewed within a self-organizing perspective, the conceptual framework provided by script theory (Abelson, 1981; Carlson, 1981; Carlson & Carlson, 1984; Tomkins, 1978, 1987) offers very interesting integrative possibilities. In particular, the notions of nuclear scripts and nuclear scenes (e.g., a nuclear script as a set of ordering rules for the connection of ensembles of prototypical affect-laden scenes—nuclear scenes—continuously reordering themselves as a result of their own activity) can be used to explain how the self-referentiality of ontological knowing (stabilization and maintenance of self-boundaries) underlies any interaction between affect and cognition. To this end, the essential aspects which characterize script processing—the development of which is traceable from early infancy (Bretherton, 1984; Nelson & Ross, 1982)—can be schematized as follows:

1. Script processing draws attention to how affect and cognition, although differentiated by their means of processing data (immediacy vs. distancing), end up acquiring a specific interdependence within a self-organizing process, such as the differentiation of self-boundaries. More specifically, the ongoing activation of opponent nuclear scenes simultaneously produces an idiosyncratic perception-of-the-world conjoined to a specific pattern of self-perception ("I") which becomes recognizable as one's own self ("Me") through script processing. In other words, the psychophysiological modulation connected with fear can only be appraised by experiencing oneself endangered ("I") and recognizing fear as an emotion consistent with one's sense of continuity and distinctness from others ("Me") through the expectations, beliefs, behavior, etc., capable of being generated about the self in this mode (cf. Cicchetti & Pogge-Hesse, 1981; Izard & Buechler, 1980). In the case mentioned above of children facing rejecting parents, for example, the activating of shame/anger is appraised through a heightened experience of the feeling of being

apart and ordered in the ongoing sense of self through the generation of consistent cognitions (low lovableness and self-worth) and behavior (avoidant attachment). It is hence possible to say that during the maturational stages, bordering the "Me" out of the perceived "I" is a process by which the immediacy of one's experience of self and the world is transformed into basic categories of meaning (self-identity, truth–falsity, competence–control, etc.), that is, into core ordering processes capable of producing and assimilating experience (Mahoney, 1988, 1991).

2. The ordering of nuclear scenes into scripts is a self-referent process, and as such involves the construction of an image of the world with an immediate and definite feeling of uniqueness to one's being-in-it, rather than mere reproduction—both faithful and, precisely for this reason, adaptive—of important aspects of the outside world. No wonder, then, if, as Tomkins (1987) notes, one of the most characteristic peculiarities of scripts is that of being "more self-validating than self-fulfilling." Indeed, script processing is more than the fine-tuning of a strategy for coping with the critical situations abstracted in nuclear scenes; it is a self-referential device constrained to activate a pattern of emotional modulation capable of stabilizing the sense of self in the world which has unfolded from those critical situations. Hence, the avoidant attachment exhibited by children of rejecting parents stabilizes the sense of being alone in a world made up of refusals or threats thereof, and it is just this stable perception of self and of external which permits considering distance as a way of maintaining emotional reciprocity. Thus, the categories of personal meaning matched by core ordering processes do not reflect simply the degree of adaptive adequacy to the environment as much as the stabilization of a coherence between the explicit sense of self and the tacit patterns of self-perception underlying it.

3. Through the maturational stages, the rhythmic and oscillative activation of prototypical nuclear scripts reordering the ongoing inflow of experience gives rise to a progressive growth and to differentiation of further subsystems of scenes and related scripts. The rate and continuity of growth of nuclear scripts reflect the course of emotive-cognitive development; in other words, the emerging subsystems are the differentiation of new perceptual-affective-motoric modulations (scenes) connected to the explicit procedures for making them consistent with one's sense of continuity (scripts). Thus, even if for each child there are relatively few prototypical nuclear scripts, they bring

about the progressive and self-regulated differentiation of a range of strictly interconnected emotional tonalities which provides his or her tacit apprehensional level with an organizational unity that makes every aspect of mental processing highly personal and idiosyncratic.

The differentiation of a structured repertoire of emotional states and rules for decoding them takes place through a matching-analogical process: perceived similarity/nonsimilarity with the immediate apprehension of reality provided by nuclear activation is the self-referent procedure for ordering the ongoing flux of events (having-a-world) while preserving the continuity of one's personal experiencing (being-in-it). The same analogical procedure also applies to the capacity for self-referring which underlies the differentiation of self-boundaries: the affective modulation acompanying the tacit apprehension of similarities ("I"), continuously decoded and reordered through available explicit processes, results in a perception of reality in which the perceiver's ongoing experience is made understandable ("Me"). Constructing a world is, therefore, a matter of abstracting one's experiential basis, and the gradual structuring of mental dimensions (categories of meaning) is seen as a process of making bodily experiences understandable. This in turn explains the crucial role exerted by metaphor development in the emergence of higher levels of rationality and cognitive abilities (Smith, 1985; Johnson, 1987; Lakoff, 1987; Lakoff & Johnson, 1980; Shanon, 1987, 1988).

SELFHOOD AS A BOUNDARY-MAINTAINING SYSTEM

An emerging sense of selfhood can begin to recognize and identify itself the moment it can differentiate between an inner sense subjectively felt and an outer sense objectively experience with others. If one considers selfhood as the underlying thread in personality development, it becomes clear that it unfolds as an open-ended and spiraling process of constructions and reconstructions resulting from the ability to experience oneself as both subject and object (Habermas, 1979; Kegan, 1982). In distinguishing the most important aspects of the development of an "I"/"Me" dynamic, it will help to bear in mind both the sequence of essential steps in ascending to more integrated levels of subject–object differentiation, and the mechanisms of systemic coherence that result once these differentiations have been produced.

The differentiation between self and others that occurs with early self-recognition (first to second year) has mainly physical characteristics, and is essentially concentrated on the immediate experience of the body (Broughton, 1978; Damon & Hart, 1982). The emerging awareness of the distinctness of others' physical appearance is oscillating and unstable for rather long periods; the edges of caregivers' boundaries slip in and out of the infant's attention, with consequent changes in his or her self-perception. Moreover, from an "others'-perspective-taking" ability rooted in physical dimensions, the infant is hardly able to differentiate between self and the rest of the body; he or she makes no clear distinction between inner and outer experiences, and the sense of self is scarcely demarcated from the swift stream of events and related feelings in which it is embedded.

Even though it diminishes because of progressive availability of concrete abstraction, this blurred differentiation continues to exist through the preschool years, making it possible for the sense of self, while gradually stabilizing, to remain bound to key perceptual features of ongoing attachments. The presence, during ontogeny, of an oscillating period preceding the stable awareness of self as demarcated from others' distinctness is probably important in modulating and further articulating the child's ability to attune, increasing empathic capabilities much more than would be the case if the sense of others were attained suddenly (Hoffman, 1984). However, it is clear that in the presence of distorted patterns of attachment, a period of loose demarcation from the perceived emotional attitudes of caregivers can also become one of critical vulnerability in the acquisition of an integrated sense of continuity and individuality. Behavior which from an external observer's viewpoint seems simply nonadaptive has a self-organizing function if looked at as a way of maintaining the internal coherence of the child. This is the case with avoidant children, whose particular kind of attachment, although matched by a negative sense of self, in practice reduces the extent of painful, disrupting emotions, establishing an emotional distance between the self and those who may hurt it.

The shifting from physical to psychological differentiation between self and others usually occurs in early childhood (ages 6–7), when others' distinctness is perceived in terms of psychological and emotional attitudes, and is matched by an increasing appreciation of one's subjectivity, felt as unique and continuous in time. By now the child clearly recognizes differences between inner and outer states, becoming able to more accurately demarcate imagination from perception, as well as to perceive psychological experiences as logically different from actual behavior.

The emerging awareness of the difference between one's inner experience ("I") and one's outer appearance ("Me") has some relevant consequences on self-boundary dynamics. As soon as the child becomes aware of having privileged access to his or her immediate experiencing, the sense of being an independent agency appears, and conscious deception becomes a real possibility for controlling relationships with significant others. Paralleling the growth in cognitive and motoric competence, the ability to actively manipulate the emotional modulation immediately experienced ("I") to maintain one's appraisal of self ("Me") as consistent increases notably because of the new possibility of self-deception now available (Buck, 1984; Damon & Hart, 1982; Habermas, 1979).

The triggering of specifically perturbing emotions (e.g., anger or helplessness in avoidant children) is short-circuited by selectively excluding sensory inflow coming from critical experiential domains. The excluding capacity obviously depends on the degree of available cognitive abilities. In young children, excluding procedures are mainly direct, and inflow, though registered, is not consciouly appraised. This type of direct exclusion is limited because covert facial motor patterns of the "true" emotional tonality that has been registered still promote some experiencing of that emotion (Campos & Caplovitz Barrett, 1984). Therefore, young children's immediacy constrains their flexibility and makes them more vulnerable to complex, ambiguous situations, whereas older children's excluding procedures, being much more indirect and mediated by semantic understanding, are more effective in changing the direction and reference of perturbing feelings.

Furthermore, whenever a child is faced with intense and not easily avoidable situations, excluding procedures become much more involved with an active manipulation on current levels of self-monitoring and awareness. One of the first modalities is that of disconnecting the perceived affect from the interpersonal situation that triggered it (Bowlby, 1980, 1985; Bretherton, 1985). When the disconnection is complete, one's experience ("I") seems completely unintelligible in terms of one's reactions ("Me") and can be better explained by attributing it to external causes such as somatic or psychological complaints. A second modality is that of preventing the appraisal of the perturbing affect from activating other feelings, thoughts, and behavior that may change one's focus of attention. In this way, children may busy themselves with many different diversionary activities (sometimes in the form of clear-cut symptoms, such as rituals, phobias, overeating, etc.) that divert them from further processing the information that, although registered, is being excluded (Bowlby, 1980, 1985). It is thus evident that exclusion of information and diversionary activity selectively constrain the elaboration of a very personal range of appraisable emotions (the only ones the child can recognize as his or her own) matched by a repertoire of automatic cognitive-emotional reactions which, by manipulating the focus of attention, allow the stabilization of such a range. Hence, throughout childhood, the self-regulating core of affective continuity—structured during preschool years as an epigenetic boundary-maintaining system—constructs from moment to moment its developmental pathway on the basis of contingencies deriving from its own pattern of internal coherence.

Finally, along with the development of reflexive abstraction occurring during adolescence, there emerges a further level of self-referring, that is, the self's awareness of its own self-awareness (Selman, 1980), and the regulative mechanisms of the boundary-maintaining system themselves become reflexive. Since the subject is able to take the perspective of the other toward him- or herself and simultaneously neutralize his or her own and the other's perspective from the third-person point of view (Dobert, Habermas, & Nunner-Winkler, 1987), one's appraisal of the self ("Me") is relatively independent from others' feedback, and so self-deceptive mechanisms maintaining consistency in one's immediate experience ("I") depend more and more on life values and philosophical axioms elaborated by the subject. In other words, the stabilization of a definite sense of self ("Me") can no longer be secured only through the level of confirmation/disconfirmation deriving from living relationships, but has to be secured reflectively, that is, through a commitment toward life embodying the uniqueness of one's being a person ("I").

3

The Self-Organization of Personal Meaning Dimensions

AN ONTOLOGICAL PERSPECTIVE

If the ordering of our world is inseparable from our being in it, then knowing corresponds to existing, and meaning is the way in which existing becomes apprehensible. Far from being a correspondence between individual beliefs and external reality which concerns almost exclusively the realm of language and abstract thought, meaning belongs primarily to the whole self-organizing activity of a human being. In other words, meaning is an *ontological understanding* in which the perceived recursiveness of one's ongoing affective-physiological modulation is consistently recognized and appraised as unitary and continuous in time through the structuring of basic categories (self-identity, truth–falsity, competence–control, etc.) of exchange between self and world able to produce and assimilate coherent experiences (Johnson, 1987; Olafson, 1988; Shanon, 1987, 1988). The qualitative aspects of this search for internal coherence are constrained by the interactional nature of human experience, where any sense of self is matched by the experience of being part of others' awareness; within an intersubjective dimension in which others support our identity, in order to feel ourselves as consistent, we have, in some way, to perceive our identity as positive enough to be supported. Indeed it seems probable that, with the emergence of abstract reflexive abilities, the primate tendency to strive for high social rank, subject to specific pressures resulting from the availability of new dimensions of intersubjectivity, had evolved into corresponding levels of reflexive self-referentiality, namely, the need to maintain self-esteem. The emerging properties of neocortical processing allowed the observer to be represented to him- or herself according to others' points of view (as perceived by the observer), and this in turn made possible a new appraisal of one's social rank in terms of more abstract self-evaluations (Barkow, 1975, Buss, 1987, 1988; Passingham, 1982; Reynolds, 1981). Striving for an acceptable self-image becomes crucial in ontological understanding, regulating both the process of making one's appraisal of self consistent and unitary and of scaffolding the experiences on which such appraisal rests.

If we start from this premise, it will be evident that any individual knowing system should be regarded, ontologically, as a self-regulating organization of personal meaning processes. Because the capacity of reflexive self-referring makes the ongoing, tacit experiencing consistent, selfhood and personal meaning come to be inextricably interwoven. Thus, consciousness, as the immediate experience of one's self, is simultaneously matched by the perception of one's being the causal agent of such experience, thereby inevitably affecting the ongoing set of possibilities in the current living context. There is no conscious experience without the influence of categories of causal attribution and self-responsibility. Moreover, the immediate experience of one's self includes a positive or negative affective modulation (perceived as a feeling of lovableness/unlovableness), and is appraised and made consistent through specific categories of self-esteem. Given that self-esteem is, as we have seen, the way in which we seek to make our conscious self-image suitable for support by others, we are justified in expecting that, in general, a perceived unlovableness corresponds to more rigorous criteria of self-esteem and vice versa. In other words, any differentiation of self-boundaries implies an ontological understanding (how far the "Me" is able to appraise its experiencing "I") in which personal meaning represents proactive processing: an ongoing ordering of networks of related meaningful events that brings forth a perception of the world capable of triggering recursive patterns of emotional modulation ("I") specifically recognizable as one's own self ("Me"), unified and continuous in time.

By means of this proactive nature, personal meaning development appears as a spiraling, open-ended process through which the essential tension inherent in selfhood dynamics unfolds: the acting and experiencing "I" is always one step ahead of the current appraisal of the situation—making it possible to perceive more than one experi-

ences, and to experience more than one attends to (Dennet, 1978)—
thus transforming the "Me" into a continuous process of reordering
and reshaping one's conscious self-image. This endless processing
(linearly exemplified by Mead's [1934] affirmation that "the 'I' of this
moment is present in the 'Me' of the next moment") resembles a kind
of "infinite game," that is, a game which, following its own rules in
an internal temporal dimension distinct from the social-objective dimension, is played not so much to win, but to continue playing
(Davis, 1983; Eigen & Winkler, 1981). We can thus confidently
state that the irreducibility of the "I"/"Me" dynamics—with its inherent proactive understanding—works as a basic push-and-pull,
and consequently the progressive unfolding of personal meaning
processes constrains the generative directionality of any individual
lifespan.

If ontologically the human way of being-in-the-world is by
seeking and creating meaning (Smith, 1978a), it should be possible,
within the intersubjective dimension that constrains the invariance of
human experience, to identify a possible set of different personal
meaning organizations, in the same manner in which, for the sake of
an analogy, it is possible to identify different physical constitutions on
the basis of the morphological invariance of the human body. Hence,
an ontological, process-oriented approach to the person should lead
us, in the final analysis, to a kind of science of meaning with an
inherent grammar of composition and recombination that can permit
the classification of the various patterns of organized coherence exhibited by people in their search for and creation of meaning.

The self-referent processes underlying the ordering of a *personal
meaning organization* (P.M.Org.) can be outlined as follows:

A P.M.Org. should not be interpreted as an *entity* defined by a
specific knowledge *content* (e.g., beliefs), but instead as a *unitary
ordering process* in which continuity and internal coherence are sought
in the specificity of the formal, structural properties of its knowledge
processing (i.e., flexibility, generativity, and abstracting level), rather
than in the definite semantic properties of its knowledge *products*.
This leads to the adoption of a systems/process-oriented methodology
that can identify the deep syntactic rules ("I") capable of generating a
consistent range of surface, semantic representations ("Me") according to an ever-changing interaction with the world. In this way, the
essential tension of selfhood as a whole would be found in the focus of
the observer's attention and, consequently, the way in which the

"Me" can recognize and make the perceived "I" consistent would become the unifying ordering process that coherently organizes patterns of affective, motor, and cognitive activity.

The self-ordering of different patterns of organizational unity of the emotional domain—structured on the basis of different developmental pathways—underlies the unfolding of correspondingly different P.M.Orgs. The next section of this chapter will outline four P.M.Orgs.: the "depressive," the "phobic," the "obsessive–compulsive," and the "eating disorders." In the experience of psychotherapy over the last 20 years these have proved to be the most typical and frequent (see Guidano, 1987; Guidano & Liotti, 1983). In each of these, the early array of nuclear scripts (as the initial unfolding of a specific developmental pathway) gives rise, in the course of maturational stages, to basic categories of personal meaning (self-identity, truth–falsity, etc.) which, starting from adolescent reflective abstraction, brings forth a scaffolding of reality that can produce supportive evidence for one's ongoing appraisal of self and world.

Naturally, further research in this direction, including describing many subsystems within each meaning dimension, will in all probability reveal some other basic dimensions of personal meaning. The point I wish to make, however, is that the number of possible basic P.M.Orgs. should be relatively small, probably between four and six, at most nine or ten. Indeed, if we assume that personal meaning reflects the pattern of emotional and psychophysiological organization, and we bear in mind the relatively small number of fundamental emotions that human beings can experience (Ekman, Levenson, & Friesen, 1983), we can see how the possibilities for combination and recombination which can produce reliable self-perception matched by an acceptable level of self-esteem must be rather small. In other words, in the face of the ever-changing multiplicity and variability of possible environmental disturbances, a differentiated set of P.M.Orgs. represents the self-referent modalities through which human consciousness comes to order that multiplicity and variability in a way which is consistent with its experience of living. This self-organizing ability for achieving coherence in a dynamic environment (in which the context for stability is continuously changing) is found from the very first stages of selfhood differentiation. For example, Main, Kaplan, and Cassidy (1985) have emphasized that, leaving aside the multiplicity and variability of possible parental attitudes, it has so far been possible to outline, quite reliably, three patterns of early central

attachment. Once more, if early central organizations are the expressions of the self-regulative and self-organizing ability of attachment processes, then these too are finite and limited in number.
Indeed, the recombinatorial possibilities between emotional modules
that can produce an emotional reciprocity, which in turn guarantees
an acceptable level of intersubjective experience, are also necessarily
reduced.

On the basis of these premises and referring the reader to
previous works for a more detailed treatment (Guidano, 1987; Guidano & Liotti, 1983), we now provide an outline of the essential features
(e.g., patterns of early reciprocity, self-boundary differentiation, "I"/
"Me" dynamics) that characterize the developmental pathways of each
of the P.M.Orgs. mentioned above.

DEVELOPMENTAL PATHWAYS

The Depressive Organization

Patterns of Early Reciprocity

The trend of attachment relationships is punctuated by a series
of affect-laden events which lend themselves to being perceived by the
child as losses, whether they be due to actual loss of a parent or to
repeated failures to develop a secure attachment through neglect
and/or rejection by uncaring parents (Bifulco, Brown, & Harris, 1987;
Bowlby, 1980; Brown, 1982; Guidano, 1987; Parker, 1983a; Weissman et al., 1987).

As a defensive strategy in response to parental rejection, infants
usually exhibit avoidant patterns of attachment, that is, active prevention of contact with caregivers and marked reduction in the expression of both distressed affect and attachment. On the one hand,
avoidant attitudes help the infant actively exclude any processing of
information that would trigger attachment, precisely in order to pre-
vent the activation of attachment behaviors that would likely not be
met with comfort or support, thus probably arousing distress and anger
(Ainsworth, 1985; Bowlby, 1980). On the other hand, with the use of
this same attitude, the infant becomes able to selectively exclude from
conscious processing a whole set of moment-to-moment rebuffs from
uncaring parents, thereby preventing the direct expression of anger
which would make further rejection even more probable; the cogni-

tive disconnection of perceived rejections, reducing the perceived level of arousal, helps the infant keep his or her ongoing patterns of self-perception stable in proximity to an attachment figure (Main & Weston, 1982). Indeed, in the histories of avoidant children, there is an absolutely characteristic tendency to minimize the experience of distressing affect on the part of the child, and a tendency to dismiss the importance of the relationship with parents as a source of comfort and support (Cassidy & Kobak, 1988).

Thus, the experience of loneliness in avoidant infants is matched by a sort of "self-caring" attitude, on the basis of which they feel able to maintain an acceptable level of reciprocity with others only by masking, at the face-to-face level of interaction, the negative affective modulation perceived during interactions with others (Lutkenhaus, Grossman, & Grossman, 1985). This involves a whole series of inappropriate affective displays in current social situations, which, almost inevitably, result in further stabilization of just that experience of loneliness on which they depend.

Self-Boundary Organization

Whether scaffolded through real deaths or separations or through parental affectionless and uncaring attitudes, the experience of loss exerts a constructional role in organizing recurrent and stable patterns of self-perception ("I") capable of being recognized and scaffolded into a stably bordered sense of self ("Me").

Organizing the "I." The reciprocal interdependence between the perception of loss and feelings of helplessness/sadness and anger is a characteristic of the biological make-up of organisms which live in an intersubjective reality, as is the case with primates (Bowlby, 1973, 1980; Panksepp, 1988; Rosenblum & Paully, 1987; Suomi, 1984). Making basic feelings such as despair and anger appraisable through a perceptual key such as loss involves the triggering of an emotional modulation (grief) of great importance for survival and adaptation; it increases the cohesion of the group through the strengthening of existing bonds.

The centrality of the loss experience during early infancy will be reflected in the selective differentiation and assembling of prototypical scenes—abstracted from events and situations repeatedly experienced—recursively oscillating between opponent emotional polarities such as helplessness/sadness and anger. By the age of 3, therefore, a recursively oscillating set of nuclear scenes begins to stabilize. Its rhythmic oscillation is able, on the one hand, to generate a quality of self-perception matched by specific psychophysiological reactions (continual alternation between anger/acting out and sadness/ withdrawal) and, on the other hand, to self-regulate through the recurrent activation of its opponent emotional tonalities (contact → anger → sadness → contact). Given that prototypical nuclear scenes become basic ingredients of infantile consciousness, the emerging "I" conveys an irreducible and immediate self-feeling which reflects the infant's experience of "being-in-the-world" (i.e., being alone in an utterly unreliable and uncontrollable world in which efforts and outcomes are perceived as unrelated); moreover, the maintenance of this inner sense through rhythmic opponent regulation cannot be experienced otherwise than through a continual succession of brusque upheavals, both within the self and in the surrounding reality.

Bordering the "Me." Given that self-recognizability is made possible through the empathic ability to take the attitudes of significant others on oneself, the profile of the "Me" that comes to be bordered invariably corresponds to a negative self-image where lovableness and personal worth are deeply underestimated. The experience of finding oneself at the center of dramatic upheavals is self-referred through the perception of one's being the causal agent of such experiences. Thus, on the one hand, the structuring of categories of internal causal attribution and self-responsibility in an attempt to tame a reality that defies control is matched by helplessness/sadness modulation; on the other hand, through the resulting anger and self-blaming attitude, it is possible to recover at least part of this control by concentrating on the negative aspects of self in order to circumscribe them. The infant's self-esteem thus coincides with the ability to make an effort to correct his or her perceived negativity and in this way maintain acceptable contact with others. The concomitant experience of loneliness also adds a sense of having to rely on oneself, both in the struggle against one's negative self, and in exploring the unknown surrounding world ("compulsive self-reliance"; Bowlby, 1977).

In these cases, rapid oscillations between anger/acting out and helplessness/withdrawal, accompanied by corresponding variations in self-esteem perception and self-blaming attitudes are practically the rule in the first part of preschool years, as though reality could be understood only through a series of alternating rejection and anger reactions. In the early years of childhood (ages 6–7), paralleling the growth in cognitive and motoric competence, the ability to actively manipulate the immediacy of emotional modulation ("I") in order to keep the appraisal of self ("Me") consistent enables the child to actively center on intermediate emotional modulation so as to avoid exposure to sudden upheavals, while still confirming and stabilizing the current sense of self. Hence, as empathetic abilities improve, shame, as the empathetic or vicarious experience of another's rejection of the self, gradually becomes a more continuous and pervasive emotional tonality, increasing the child's sensitivity to criticism, contempt, and rejection, and thus also the possibility of anticipating them (Izard & Schwartz, 1986; Lewis, 1986, 1988). From the second stage of childhood on, the child stabilizes around steady patterns of self-perception by keeping the range of perceived rejections or failures fairly constant through a series of self-deceptive, decentralized controls. The avoidant style, which permits reduction in the emotional arousal resulting from interpersonal events, is accompanied by an even more selective and efficient exclusion of critical inflow from the significant interpersonal domain. In addition, the repertoire of diversionary activities permits a certain degree of control over anger, thus further reducing the possibilities of rejection or failure. For example, the frequency of self-injuries (also reported in separated monkeys; Suomi, 1984), apart from averting one's own anger away from others, also works as an emotional self-stimulus within a situation which mimics the features of partial sensory deprivation.

The developmental pathway that emerges is one in which the continuous anticipation of loss by the helpless child is, at the same time, the self-referent process for confirming and stabilizing one's ongoing sense of being-in-the-world and the most effective way of reducing the intensity of disruptive emotions from losses and rejections, which in turn are perceived as certain and inevitable.

From the end of puberty and paralleling the emergence of new levels of reflexive self-referring, the internal causal attribution that characterizes the "Me" and the struggle to overcome negativity expand considerably throughout adolescence and youth, becoming more and more abstract and independent of the immediate emotional context, giving rise to a more articulated and inclusive way of ordering reality.

"I"/"Me" Dynamics and Systemic Coherence

Selfhood dynamics in depressive meaning rest on the essential tension between the pervasive and immediate scaffolding of the world in terms of losses, rejections, and failures ("I") and explicit reordering of the world in terms of a negative self and internal causal attribution ("Me") as the essential self-referent strategy for consistently recognizing and appraising one's moment-to-moment experiencing.

From one point of view, the internal causal attribution underlying a negative self-image makes it possible to restore an actor's sense of being a person who is recentering the struggle for control over the self, rather than over an unreliable world. From this perspective, the depressive attributional style described by the reformulated model of learned helplessness in which uncontrollable events are attributed to characteristics of the self in a stable and global way (Abramson, Seligman, & Teasdale, 1978; Seligman & Peterson, 1986) appears to be the primary self-regulatory process for preserving the internal coherence of a depressive meaning in assimilating experience. Consequently, the scaffolding of reality in terms of losses and failures should not be considered only an abnormal feature, as if it merely consisted of a sort of cumulative and passive reverberation of past schemata. On the contrary, it is an autonomous and creative knowing strategy in which generativity and novelty are based on the active construction of a growing sense of the inaccessibility of reality. Indeed, if a stable, external negative attribution were coupled with a steady emotional modulation in terms of helplessness/anger ("I"), the "Me" that would be appraisable would be perceived only as a helpless object at the mercy of an adverse, unpredictable reality; a more definite sense of the "Me" as an active agency would then become possible only through the structuring of a persecutory, frightening delusion of living in a hostile world.

From another viewpoint, the rhythmic oscillation between anger/motor activation and helplessness/motor slowing down is experienced as abrupt and contrasting changes in one's ongoing self-perception, perceived, most of the time, in rapid succession in the same situation. These perceived reversals in one's immediate experiencing are recognized and tentatively made consistent by varying the intensity and quality of the internal causal attribution to the negative self, eventually triggering equally abrupt reversals of quality (in the sense of self-esteem) in the course of a given situation. Thus, within the same situation, the immediate sense of being unlovable and worthless may be perceived as something which can be strenuously and competently fought against with the feeling that one's personal worth really depends on such a struggle (anger and motor activation). Moments later, however, the same negative traits may be perceived as intrinsic, inescapable ingredients of the self, toward which the only coherent attitude is a self-blaming one with consequent deactivation of any activity under way (helplessness and motor slowing down). This continual alternation of feeling, chosen or damned by the same destiny, so characteristic of the depressive meaning, also becomes evident, in our opinion, on the microgenetic level (cf. Draguns, 1984), when one tries, within single and discrete cognitive-emotive abilities, to trace patterns that appear in a telescoped fashion in overall lifespan development. Hence, for example, depressive people, compared to others, tend to show heightened initial reactions to emotionally significant warning stimuli, followed by withdrawal and slowing down of affective processing as the actual stimulus approaches (Yee & Miller, 1988). Similarly, during recognition trials applied to negative mood induction procedures, depressive people exhibit an alternating display of both elated and dysphoric contents (Small & Robins, 1988).

Evidently, then, the essential aspect that transforms the "I"/ "Me" dynamics of depressive meaning into an open-ended process is the fact that reordering perceived losses in terms of internal attribution is always one step behind experiencing reality in terms of losses. This is reflected in the depressive's striking tendency to bring about a series of events in his or her social and cultural network, all of which are capable of being scaffolded in terms of losses and failures. Consequently, the orthogenetic directionality that constrains the unfolding of depressive meaning should be identified (in terms of positive progression) with a continuous differentiation and integration of the loss theme, matched by a shifting of the capability for reflexive self-referring toward more and more abstract levels, to the point where the individual experiences loss as a category of human experience rather than as a personal destiny of loneliness and rejection. It goes without saying that such a point should be considered more as a kind of "ideal" normative progression rather than as an effective goal to be reached in one phase or other of the individual life cycle.

The Phobic Organization

Patterns of Early Reciprocity

Despite their diversity, the invariant aspect characterizing patterns of parental attachment consists of an *indirect* inhibition of the infant's autonomous exploratory behavior, either through overprotection or through the parents' unavailability as a safe base. As far as the infants are concerned, the invariant aspect consists of the fact that they never feel that their lovableness or personal value is put into question. In the overprotective pattern they feel their liberty of movement is restricted because they are loved too much; but it is they themselves who, because of a kind of excess of solicitousness, take the initiative in maintaining close contact with the parents, and refrain from exploring their surroundings (Arindell, Emmelkamp, Monsma, & Brilman, 1983; Bowlby, 1973, 1983, 1988; Parker, 1979, 1983b).

In other words, the indirect way in which inhibition is carried out represents the crucial variable, and consequently feeling oneself limited in one's freedom of movement can only be experienced as something that is necessarily part of an attachment relationship which can be perceived as stable and "safe" (Guidano, 1987, 1988; Guidano & Liotti, 1983, 1985). Clearly, the infant's experience of his or her being-in-the-world is specifically constrained, from the very start, by this stipulation. Indeed, on the one hand, the interference with inborn tendencies toward autonomous environmental exploration is matched by an appreciable degree of emotional distress which, further intensifying the search for proximity to an attachment figure, gives rise to a true anxious attachment; that is, the infant feels protected from the environment, perceived as dangerous, only when in close physical contact with a caregiver (clinging attitude). On the other hand, the indirectness of such interference prevents the infant from perceiving the distress as coming from parents' intentions concerning upbringing, and therefore as something referable to his or her own emotional attitudes or qualities, and so the child is unable to localize it inside his or her emerging subjective experience. As a consequence, the emotional distress is experienced as localized in the physical aspects of the self, and the infant becomes able to control it by selectively excluding any arousal modulation which, regardless of its emotional content, would exceed his or her perceived range of stability.

Nonetheless, controlling embodied distress by excluding any arousal modulation is paralleled by a pervasive feeling of low competence in managing one's emotional states. All this would lead to a further reduction in the perceived range of stability were it not counterbalanced by an overcontrolling attitude toward the environment which excludes any initiative that would decrease the proximity from a protective figure by perceiving any possible novelty as a potential danger. It follows that an attitude of this kind brings with it a continual reproduction of feelings of constriction and limitation, ending with the stabilization of the experience of an endangered and distressed self on which it depends.

Self-Boundary Organization

Within a developmental pathway characterized by overcontrol of distress perceived through the body, selfhood differentiation is carried out through somewhat specific patterns.

Organizing the "I." The inhibition of autonomous exploration is reflected in the selective differentiation and unitary assembling of prototypical scenes in which attachment and separation, rather than regulating reciprocally and developing side by side, are experienced as situations in which one excludes the other; this is equivalent to perceiving any temporary separation from a protective figure as an impending danger, then immediately feeling constricted and limited the moment physical contact with that same figure is re-established. So at about the age of 3, the array of recursively oscillating nuclear scenes regarding the mutal exclusion of protection and autonomy brings forth a self-regulating pattern of self-perception in which the felt need for freedom and independence is matched by the distressing perception of a dangerous world in which being lovingly protected is the only possible way to be-in-it.

Fear and distress experienced through the oscillation of body arousal become the main ingredients of the emerging "I," selectively orienting ongoing perceptive-cognitive processing toward a "sensorial" decoding of any emotional modulation in such a way as to forestall any arousal oscillation which may overreach one's perceived range of stability.

Bordering the "Me." While the subject's sense of continuity rests on the experience of controlling the modulation of arousal resulting from the rhythmic oscillation of negative emotional tonalities, that is, distress/need for protection and need for freedom/fear, overprotective parental attitudes bias self-recognizability toward a positive bordering of the "Me." Because of the capability for stabilizing one's ongoing arousal by a selective tuning to the sensorial aspects of emotional experience (i.e., feeling emotions through the body), the child becomes able to appraise him- or herself as lovable and valuable. The profile of the "Me" that emerges is one in which emotionality and effusive behavior are equated with fragility and weakness, and are consequently excluded from the perceived emotional range. Since controllable emotions are identified with controllable sensorial modulation, the dimensions of personal subjective experience are somewhat reduced from the start, and self-esteem and self-competence become closely related to self-control. This appraisal of the self is made consistent by attributing the felt need for protection to a stable, negative external cause (i.e., an "objectively" dangerous world) and explaining one's overcontrolling attitude in terms of the need for freedom and independence.

As childhood progresses, the child becomes more able to keep within an acceptable range any discrepant modulation of arousal connected to frightening experiences of loneliness (need for protection) and constriction (need for freedom). Orienting attention on the sensorial cues of feelings and refraining from further processing other aspects of emotionality relevant to his or her subjectivity, the child can achieve a dynamic and steady equilibrium through specific patterns of self-deceptive, decentralized control by: (1) progressively excluding all sensory inflow capable of activating the need for freedom and independence which would invariably trigger loneliness distress; and (2) structuring a repertoire of somatic and visceral complaints that act as diversionary activity for maintaining proximity to protective figures without having to decode it as a constriction.

Consequently, in a developmental pathway of this kind, many ensembles of affect-laden nuclear scripts are not properly reordered and transformed into semantic cognitive content. The activation of these scripts is likely to be expressed through arousal-motor patterns of reaction, and this further stabilizes the existing trend of referring one's emotions to perceived bodily modifications. Fear and distress thus remain the most structured and easily recognizable feelings within one's perceived emotional range, making it indispensable to seek proper self-control through the achievement of secure proximity to protective figures.

Finally, from adolescence on, the emergence of new levels of reflexive self-referring allows for a more abstract reordering of the "Me" overcontrolling attitude. The rhythmic oscillation of opponent emotional experiences ("I") is matched by a sense of being a controlling agent ("Me"), and the attitude appraised as either self-reliance—if based upon confirmation of one's ability to find other available protective figures in every possible new circumstance (need for protection)—or as autonomy and independence—if based on confirmation of one's ability to control interpersonal relationships able to provide an adequate sense of protection (need for freedom).

"I"/"Me" Dynamics and Systemic Coherence

Phobic selfhood dynamics rest on the essential tension between the pervasive and immediately experienced need to rely on secure, affective relationships ("I") and the explicit reordering in terms of a controlling agent ("Me") which renders the individual unable to master the existential and emotional aspects inherent in the human affective domain.

On the one hand, an explicit self-image whose positivity relies on emotional overcontrol and exclusion entails the tendency to assume an external attributive attitude toward one's immediate experiencing, in which feelings and emotions are regarded as external to the self. Controlling procedures are therefore based on an almost automatic prevention or avoidance of emotions, rather than on their understanding in terms of personal meaning (Guidano, 1987, 1988; Guidano & Liotti, 1985).

On the other, the rhythmic oscillation between distress/need for protection and need for freedom/fear implies a tendency to overreact with high emotional intensity to variations, even minimal, in one's affectional balance. This may occur particularly in reaction to threats of detachment (however imaginary) from protective figures, and conversely, to any increase in emotional involvement in an ongoing affective relationship which may be perceived as a limitation of one's freedom of action. However, the same overcontrolling attitude makes the "Me" blind to the emotions being experienced ("I"), to the point where they can be felt only as physical distress, either as a need for protection or as a fear of constriction. It is well known, in fact, that whenever there are difficulties in using appropriate cognitive scaffolding to decode one's ongoing emotional modulation, the latter is usually experienced as alien, negative, and more or less painful (Bowlby, 1985; Marshall & Zimbardo, 1979; Maslach, 1979).

It is thus evident that the generativity of phobic "I"/"Me" dynamics lies precisely in the attempt to control an emotion, to the point where it is excluded from the explicit self-image, but only after this same emotion has actually been experienced. Making new affective bonds, breaking old ones, or perceiving growing loneliness or constriction in significant relationships can easily trigger emotional experiences whose control would require more complex self-explanations than those allowed by the ongoing controlling attitude. However, through the assimilation and integration of such disequilibria, a phobic meaning can undergo a progressive differentiation of the perceived range of personal emotions and eventually reach more articulated and comprehensive balances between its central, opposing needs.

The Eating Disorders Organization

Patterns of Early Reciprocity

Despite their diversity from one case to the next, attachment relationships are characterized by certain invariant aspects which concur to trigger a specific experience in the child's unfolding selfhood by combining together into a unitary sequence in the course of maturation (Guidano, 1987, 1988). Parental attachment style is usually ambiguous and undefined, and generally contradictory. On the one hand, they portray themselves as parents completely devoted to the well-being and upbringing of their children; on the other, their parenting behavior is more concerned with obtaining confirmation of that image from others than with fulfilling their children's concrete need for emotional warmth and support. Hence, mothers, although very concerned with the infant, derive no pleasure from nursing, and self-control prevails over caring and tenderness (Selvini-Palazzoli, 1978). This maternal selective inattention to the infant's cues results in interference in the rhythmic and synchronic patterns of reciprocal attunement right from the beginning of mother–infant dyadic interaction (Chatoor, 1989; Chatoor, Egan, Getson, Menvielle, & O'Don-

nell, 1988). Difficulty in abstracting meaningful self-referent regularities from caregivers' behavior prevents the infant from scaffolding his
or her sensory inflow into an organized stream of recurrent psychophysiological rhythms. Apart from the primitive bodily rhythms
connected with hunger and motility, many others remain deregulated
and desynchronized, since adequate interconnections with basic feelings and motor patterns cannot be established. Consequently, self-
recognition processes can only give rise to a blurred sense of self, and,
given the parents' essential upbringing strategy of constant anticipation or redefinition of the infant's feelings, the child easily develops a
deep and pervasive feeling of unreliability in recognizing his or her
ongoing inner states. Various factors (rhythm deregulation, intrusive
parenting, etc.) interfere with the emergent perception of being an
entity distinct from other people, and the infant can only achieve
self-recognition, and hence a reasonably stable pattern of self-
perception, through an enmeshed relationship with an attachment
figure (Minuchin, 1974; Minuchin, Rosman, & Baker, 1978).

Given that the child, in order to achieve a stable, definitive
sense of self, must comply with the expectations of an attachment
figure perceived as an absolute model, any reappraisal of that figure
can obviously only be experienced as a disappointment—one so intense as to call into question his or her already established self-image.
In this way, the "physiological" change of parents' image (i.e., relativization resulting from more abstract conceptual perspective-taking)
which comes with the maturation of reflexive cognitive abilities again
triggers the emergence of a blurred and wavering immediate experiencing, making the achievement of a stable sense of self problematic. However, since an enmeshed relationship with a significant
figure remains the essential strategy for obtaining a definitive self-
image, the problem now becomes one of finding reliable partners
without risking further possible disappointments and failures.

Self-Boundary Organization

In a developing situation characterized by a poor demarcation
between self and others, selfhood differentiation can be outlined as
follows.

Organizing the "I." The deregulation/desynchronization of early
rhythms is paralleled by a relatively undifferentiated patterning of

psychophysiological modulation, giving rise to a pervasive and distressing blurred experiencing of self. Moreover, the rehearsal of nuclear scenes concerning the nonrecognition or disconfirmation of any expression of autonomous feelings and thoughts brings about the selective structuring of opponent sets of prototypical scenes, all rather undifferentiated and loosely interconnected. As a result, the immediate self-feeling is continuously wavering between the experience of being "externally bound" in recognizing one's internal states (in which the obtained sense of individuality is matched by a sense of personal ineffectiveness) or the experience of being "internally bound" in defining one's ongoing emotional modulation (in which the perceived stronger sense of individuality is intermingled with a feeling of emptiness and self-unreliability). Thus, personal ineffectiveness and a sense of emptiness, continuously triggered by wavering self-experiencing, become the main ingredients of the emerging "I," and, as the infant's attention selectively attunes to interpersonal cues, eventually give rise to an overreliance upon external frames of reference.

Bordering the "Me." The reordering of one's immediate experience into a definite sense of self is carried out according to external frames of reference. Self-recognizability therefore eventually coincides with perceived expectations of an attachment figure, and the profile of the "Me" is reflected by the corresponding self-image able to fit with such expectations. Hence, if the problem consists of drawing a definite sense of self out of others' attitudes and judgments, perfectionism becomes the way to provide an optimal solution to this problem. As a consequence, the "Me" is framed according to standards of perfection, as absolute as they are conventional, and the attempt to achieve them is considered the most reliable way of attaining an acceptable level of self-esteem and self-worthiness.

The quality of the appraisal of disappointment, while restricting one's range of self-exposure and self-confrontation, defines the prevailing orientation of causal attribution (i.e., external vs. internal), even though such orientation, stemming from a blurred and wavering immediate experience, remains within loose, vague margins. Whether an external rather than internal orientation will prevail depends on the extent to which the appraisal of the prototypical disappointment is actively "discovered" (i.e., experienced as the result of one's own activity) as opposed to being passively "accepted" (i.e., experienced coercion to adapt to an overwhelming distressing event) (Beattie-Emery & Csikszentmihalyi, 1981; Guidano, 1987).

In the case of an external orientation, the "Me" perceives others mainly as deceitful and intrusive; striving against a deceitful reality by strenuously displaying positive, controlled, self-sufficient attitudes becomes the essential means for keeping the pervasive feeling of ineffectiveness and emptiness below acceptable limits. This attributional style, which involves more active bodily and motoric patterns, can give rise, whenever unbalanced, to typical anorexic disorders.

In the case of internal orientation, however, the "Me" will be focused on restricting the distressing effect of expected disconfirmations by attributing them to specific, concrete traits of the self, rather than to feelings of personal ineffectiveness and emptiness that pervade one's immediate experiencing. Whenever unbalanced, this attributional style, involving more passive bodily and motoric patterns, can be the source of bulimic disorders and obesity.

Hence, from the end of childhood on, a blurred and wavering "I" is reordered into a self-image whose competence and worthiness depend on the equilibrium which one has been able to establish between the absolute need for significant others' approval and the impending fear of being intruded upon or disappointed in significant relationships. On the one hand, adhering to absolute standards associated with everyday common sense brings forth an image of the self as reliable and worthy because of the perceived ability to manipulate others' judgment in one's own favor. On the other hand, avoiding self-exposure and self-confrontation allows the recovery of individuality and demarcation from others in one's self-image because of the perceived ability to control the intrusiveness and deceitfulness of others.

Clearly an attitude of this kind implies the selective exclusion of any inflow which is able either to interfere with the attunement to absolute standards, or to increase self-exposure, given that in both cases challenging disconfirmations of one's self-image would become more probable. Hence, the most striking feature of the eating disorders personal meaning is the vague and continually oscillating attitude of the "Me" toward the "I"; that is, the oscillative and uncertain attribution of causality with respect to one's feelings and inner modulation self-regulates in such a way that the perfectionist attitude is buffered against disconfirmations by the parallel structuring of very specific self-deceiving patterns. Both the attributive oscillation and the overreliance on external frames of reference, in fact, make it possible for perceived feelings to emerge in consciousness as loosely and vaguely interconnected with other concurrent emotions, images, and conscious thoughts. This capability for managing different and often contrasting aspects of consciousness by not connecting them in turn prevents the "Me" from becoming completely aware of what the "Me" itself actually knows. In this manner, a variety of possibilities open up for self-manipulative mechanisms designed to maintain one's perceived self-esteem; for example, it then becomes possible to assert from moment to moment either that one feels prey to fear or that one never experiences fear because of one's willpower. All this, moreover, is not even perceived as a discrepancy, given that, rather than making ongoing immediate experience consistent, it is the moment-to-moment search for a "coherence of appearance" that stabilizes one's self-image. Also, the modulation of basic bodily rhythms like hunger and motility provides the only possibilities for a reliable self-perception within a continuously wavering immediate experiencing; therefore, variations in eating and motor behavior act as diversionary activities which reduce the chance of challenging feelings of emptiness and/or ineffectiveness entering consciousness.

Finally, because of the role that formal and aesthetic aspects play in a coherence of appearance, the possibility of having an unacceptable body image is the essential way of embodying feelings of ineffectiveness or emptiness once the latter have been triggered by inevitable or unpredictable confrontations. The more active anorexic pattern strives against this image of failure by overcontrolling biological impulses; the obese pattern, on the contrary, in trying to circumscribe an expected failure, tends to give up the struggle.

"I"/"Me" Dynamics and Systemic Coherence

The essential tension underlying selfhood dynamics in the eating disorders meaning is easily traceable to the problem of a loose and indefinite demarcation from others. The pervasive and compelling need for supportive intimacy in order to experience a fairly stable pattern of self-perception continuing in time ("I") is accompanied by its explicit reordering as a competent and valuable self-image ("Me") whose absoluteness, while being the perceived requisite for attaining supportive intimacy, requires a nearly total reduction of self-disclosure which eventually excludes any intimacy whatever.

Thus, in order to avoid any definite affective commitment and self-exposure—which would imply the risk of negative judgments calling into question the established standards for one's self-image—a whole repertoire of relational strategies aims at obtaining *a priori* from the partner the absolute guarantee of a supportive intimacy. However, in the rather improbable case that such an external guarantee were to be obtained in this manner, it would in no way solve the compelling need to experience an "inner-founded" self; as Pirandello put it in his famous play *Rules of the Game:* the mirror usually reflects only the way others see us, the way we are expected to behave, forced to behave— hardly ever what we really are. Thus, in most situations, an affectional style characterized by ambiguity, indefiniteness, and constant "testing" of the partner often brings about the very criticisms and disappointments which could have been avoided.

However, the assimilation and integration of such distressing feelings, triggering further reorderings of the "Me," enable it to recognize internal frames of reference in the "I" for organizing more reliable, stable patterns of self-perception. In other words, the "ideal," generative lifespan directionality of an eating disorders meaning is one in which a progressive demarcation from others, with the consequent relativization of those others, is matched by a growing sense of individuality and personal autonomy.

The Obsessive–Compulsive Organization

Patterns of Early Reciprocity

The essential feature of the organization of obsessive meaning is the unitary combination which, in the developing infant, acquires two aspects which may be considered invariant: firstly, an ongoing, immediate experience in terms of intense, antithetical feelings which increase the need for emotional/analogue processing; secondly, a primacy given to verbal/analytical processing which eventually reduces the actual possibilities of viable emotional decoding.

Parenting behavior in these cases assumes all the characteristics of a truly ambivalent "double-faced" attachment, where concealed rejecting attitudes are camouflaged by an outward facade of absolute devotion and concern. The *simultaneousness* of parents' antithetical attitudes seems to be the crucial variable, given that eventually it takes the form of a "double-bind" situation, that is, a communicative setting in which any available understanding is inevitably experienced by the infant as probably wrong (Bateson, Jackson, Haley, & Weakland, 1956; Sluzki & Veron, 1976). While the image of an apparently all-giving, overindulgent parent is matched by an emotional modulation conveying a feeling of reliability of one's being-in-the-world, the simultaneous experiencing of the same parent as demanding, controlling, and rejecting triggers an opposite emotional modulation in which one's perceived unacceptability is mixed with feelings of anger and hostility. In other words, the uncontrollability perceived by the infant could be paraphrased by saying that the experiences "He or she loves me; I'm lovable" and "He or she loves me not; I'm unlovable" both have evidence in their favor and explain equally well the same ongoing attachment relationship.

In this way, the structuring of a psychophysiological modulation characterized by abrupt and recurrent oscillations between antithetical feelings parallels the emergence of split patterns of self-recognition which, being mutually exclusive, reduce the possibility of organizing unitary patterns of self-perception. As a whole, parents' attitudes outline a highly verbal and motorically underactive intersubjective dimension (Adams, 1973), that is, an almost absolute predominance of rational explanations and analytical reasoning procedures over immediate forms of communication (positive or negative emotional exchanges, games and physical activity, spontaneity, etc.). The continual need to adhere explicitly to an established external order of rules and absolute principles gives shape to a truly unreasonably demanding environment for the child, and eventually becomes an instrument for the parents to obtain virtually total control over his or her behavior and emotions (Clark & Bolton, 1985; Salzman, 1973). Feelings and emotional expressions are eventually excluded from this established order through a characteristic procedure: not that feelings should be controlled, but rather that they are not to be felt at all. Since feelings once triggered are, by their very nature, unavoidable and inescapable, any emotional modulation is likely to be experienced by the child as a pervasive sense of uncontrollability, further stabilizing his or her orientation toward the verbal/analytical dimension.

Self-Boundary Organization

Organizing the "I." The rhythmic rehearsal of nuclear scenes concerning ambivalent situations and unresolvable dilemmas tacitly perceived is matched by recurrent and abrupt oscillations between antithetical feelings and opposite and incompatible perceptions of self. Patterns of self-recognition, structured on the basis of such oscillations, outline a "double-faced" experiencing of the self, alternately perceived as a pervasive feeling of ambivalence, or as a distressing fear of uncontrollability. Thus, ambivalence and uncontrollability, frequently surfacing as bizarre and frightening "insights" about oneself, become the main ingredients of the emerging "I," selectively attuning the infant's available resources toward a "cognitive" search for consistency/certainty and control.

Bordering the "Me." The reordering of an ambivalent and antithetical immediate experience into a definite sense of self results from the differentiation of opposite patterns of self-perception and the active selection of one of them as one's self-image. The criterion for self-recognizability thus corresponds to the perceived external established order, and the profile of the "Me" is then acceptable insofar as it manages to exclude from processing a large part of ongoing immediate experience. In other words, while, for example, a depressive "Me" is matched by a set of possible self-images relying on polarities of helplessness and anger, an obsessive "Me" is forced to rely moment-to-moment on only *one* of the polarities, that is, either he or she is lovable and acceptable, or he or she is neither. Further limited by poor growth of analogical/tacit understanding, the child becomes selectively inattentive to the emotional modulation provided by his or her immediate experiencing—preferring thought and linguistic capabilities to the point of making them the essential instrument for any understanding. In comparison to the perceivable ambivalence of images and emotions, verbal processes appear more consistent and easily controllable, as their digital-sequential format allows the distribution of information into two distinctly differentiable opposites, facilitating the selection of the right one.

Patterns of decentralized control for maintaining one's selected self-image will therefore be based on this "verbal primacy." On the one hand, the selective exclusion of free fantasy, imagery, emotions, and impulses substantially decreases the surfacing into consciousness

of ambivalent feelings; on the other, a whole repertoire of diversionary activities diverts selective attention from further processing by moment-to-moment emotional modulation. These activities take on the form of thoughts (ruminations, doubts, etc.) very often connected to stereotyped behavior (rituals), since in the concrete stage of childhood, motoric patterns are the prevailing means of controlling the unfolding of cognitive abilities.

The surfacing of mixed, ambivalent feelings, which continues to occur, is made consistent through the structuring of a "Me" opposite attitude, that is, feeling and thinking exclusively by way of opposite categories, passing from one to the other in an "all-or-none" way, so that unless the perception of certainty is matched by a sense of total control, the "Me" tends to perceive a total lack of control (Salzman, 1973). The "Me" all-or-none attitude carries out a self-referent procedure for perceiving a unitary identity out of the double-faced experiencing "I"; in any situation, in fact, an all-or-none decoding makes available a consistent and consequently certain perception of self and reality, the only difference being that in one case it will be positive, and in the other negative.

The attribution of causality will vary in an all-or-none way depending on the quality of the "Me" appraisal. In the positive dimension, an external causal attribution will prevail, and the need for certainty will be expressed by constant activity aimed at foreseeing and anticipating any possible unexpected event brought about by a deceiving, untrustworthy reality. In the negative dimension, conversely, the pervasive sense of an inherent and uncontrollable negativity of the self is the essential means by which an internal causal attribution attempts to control ambivalent and perturbing feelings triggered by ongoing discrepant experience.

Within a developmental pathway in which the certainty of one's perceived identity is acquired through the exclusion of one's emotional life, the commitment to certainty in any domain of experience becomes the essential procedure for maintaining a unitary and reliable self-perception. Because the perception of a unitary identity is equated with the perceived certainty of having total control over oneself, the overconfidence in thought, verbal fluency, and linguistic competence eventually becomes a selective attitude for maintaining the range of emotional processing within fairly narrow limits. By regarding only the rational and logical aspects of one's ongoing emotional modulation as worthy of attention and further processing, it actually becomes possible to exclude ambivalent feelings (which would call into question the selected self-image) and feelings such as hostility, anger, and sexuality, which could trigger a perturbing sense of shame, incompetence, and unworthiness.

The constant search for certainty that one has total control over oneself is matched by a perfectionist attitude resulting from the moment-to-moment adhesion to a rigid set of moral standards and rules. We are, however, dealing with a "nonspecific perfectionism," which is seldom actualized in one's ongoing life programs, for the sense of being a positive and reliable person depends almost exclusively on the *formal adherence* to moral rules perceived as absolute certainties. Being perfect thus means seeking justice, equity, and truth for their own sake, with little correlation to the irreducible unique aspects of ongoing existential situations.

The dynamic equilibrium between antithetical dimensions of controllability and uncontrollability permitted by a selfhood dynamic of this type is shored up by fairly specific self-deceiving patterns of decentralized control. As a response to unpredictable double-faced immediate experiences that split the current selected self-image into opposing positive and negative ones, the "Me" regains total control by displacing causal attribution, in an all-or-none way, toward an internally perceived negativity. This attributional shift temporarily dislocates these opposing self-images, so that the negative "actual" self is matched by the positivity of a "potential" self perceived as possible in the near future (Makhlouf-Norris & Norris, 1972). In other words, the "Me" can maintain a negative but certain identity in actuality, while at the same time preventing self-esteem from decreasing to below acceptable limits.

"I"/"Me" Dynamics and Systemic Coherence

The essential tension underlying selfhood dynamics would thus seem to be traceable to a deeply ingrained emotional imbalance (dichotomous experiencing of the "I") reflected in the struggle to attain a unitary and reliable perception of one's self-image ("Me"). In a situation in which a steady double-bind attachment is the basis for the undecodability of one's feelings, thought processes—in their concrete and, subsequently, abstract forms—are the only possible avenue for reaching a unitary and reliable perception. In other words, the antithetical opposition between thinking and feeling, which emerges as a result of a structural discrepancy in the "Me" appraisal of the "I," is central to the organization of obsessive meaning, being at the same time the source of a whole set of specific perturbations which may, at any moment, prejudice the equilibrium it has attained.

On the one hand, the search for certainty carried out solely through cognitive modes is matched by the tendency to split up ongoing experience, dwelling excessively on its constituent details and failing to envisage the whole ("underinclusion"; Reed, 1969, 1985). The relative incapacity to reach integrated perspectives depends both on the selective omission of global apprehensional frames (i.e., images) supplied by the ongoing emotional modulation, and on the rigid dichotomization of any experience into opposing aspects, to be certain of pursuing the positive aspects and carefully avoiding the negative ones. Systematic doubting becomes the preferred strategy for reaching a unitary and stable experiencing of reality, and the resulting pedantic attitude is, usually, in keen contrast to the individual's linguistic and rhetorical abilities. Doubting, procrastination, and overconcern for details will therefore prevail whenever the situation to be faced presents some complexity, reaching the point where, in the most intense situations, the ability to make a decision is lost. The perceived difficulty in deciding about something highly thought of and valued is, in turn, one of the immediate experiences that is most likely to trigger pervasive and ambivalent feelings, whose emergence into consciousness would call into question the currently selected self-image.

On the other hand, while a positive and emotionally "clear" affective involvement would represent a possible source of nonambivalent reciprocity, allowing for better decoding and reordering of one's double-faced experiencing, the possibilities of genuine involvement are reduced, since all the sense of unity and continuity depends on the perception of having total control over oneself. Quite the contrary, as mentioned, it is precisely the affective situations (making and breaking affectional bonds, pregnancy, childbirth, etc.) which turn out to be the most complex, and the most difficult about which to make a decision. Furthermore, because the control of emotions is directed at the rigid exclusion of any emotional-imaginative modulation, the individual has a tendency to experience even the slightest feelings that escape his or her control as extremely intense, with a consequent tendency to overreact unduly. The possibility of perceiving oneself as being at the mercy of one's own emotions is in turn matched by a pervasive and distressing sense of uncontrollability intermingled with other challenging feelings, such as shame, guilt, and unworthiness.

The intermittent emergence of uncontrollable feelings that challenge the reliability of one's self-image and subsequent attempts to assimilate and integrate them are at the core of the generativity and orthogenetic progression exhibited by an obsessive meaning. The resulting directionality should be expressed in the course of lifespan development by a progressive relativization of the image of an absolute and certain reality, matched by the emergence of an irreducible sense of one's uniqueness based on a more adequate decoding of one's emotional modulation. In other words, the switching in meaning level, which proves to be crucial in an obsessive lifespan, consists of the existential discovery that the sense of a sure identity cannot rely on the impersonal universality of thought, but rather on the perceived uniqueness of one's personal emotional domain.

METHODOLOGICAL IMPLICATIONS FOR PSYCHOPATHOLOGY

The ontological perspective that has been sketched out up to this point demands a drastic revision of the methodological program underlying current notions in clinical psychology and psychopathology. I shall limit myself to a few considerations on two essential points: (1) the necessity of a process-oriented, explicative psychopathology which can take into account classes of behavior perceived as clinical disturbances by an external observer; and (2) a reformulation in terms of systems/process-oriented principles of current conceptualization concerning mental health and mental disorders.

Explanatory Psychopathology as a Science of Meaning

The basic ambiguity regarding current clinical methodology—as exemplified, for instance, by DSM-III-R—lies in the fact that it is (1) essentially atheoretical, and (2) merely descriptive (Faust & Miner, 1986; Weimer, 1979, 1984).

1. In trying to be an exemplifcation of the empiricist principle of parsimony (i.e., remaining as close to the "data" as possible) an

atheoretical clinical approach has in the end encouraged professional acceptance of an almost total ignorance of etiology and psychopathological processes, which, in fact, should be the essential motivation for their research. This ignorance is the expression of a methodological choice: avoiding any investigation of the etiological problem. This choice emerges in full measure when the DSM-III-R invites psychiatric clinicians to agree on the identification of mental disorders on the basis of clinical manifestations without even agreeing on how those disorders occur. We are dealing with a situation which is becoming more and more evident and often embarrassing, as recent data concerning the involvement of psychologists and psychiatrists in the legal arena attest. Evidence indicates that professionals often fail to reach reliable or valid conclusions, and the accuracy of their judgments does not necessarily surpass that of laypersons, thus raising substantial doubt that psychologists or psychiatrists meet legal standards for expertise (Faust & Ziskin, 1988).

It should be clear that the renunciation of etiological understanding excludes, in real terms, the possibility of establishing what relationship there may be between observed behavior and the organization of the person who exhibits it. It is therefore natural that the planning of treatment is the result of guesswork. All this, which at first glance might seem a little paradoxical, like planning the decor of a house one has not seen, corresponds to attitudes as ingrained as they are accepted, given that it has been possible to prepare techniques for modifying "erroneous" knowledge without stopping to ask how that knowledge arises.

On the other hand, if, using the perspective we have been presenting, we put ourselves in the position of the individual who self-organizes his or her knowledge, it would seem to follow that we should accept the fact that the only adequate etiological understanding is that of a developmental psychopathology, that is, the multilevel reconstruction of lifespan transformational experiences which bring about the patterns of meaning coherence exhibited at present by the individual. Rather than being random or totally empirical, as empiricist postulates would require, such a reconstruction can be understood through a developmental theory that appreciates the complexity of adaptational processes as well as the regularity through which basic transformations are carried out (Bowlby, 1988; Guidano, 1987; Mahoney, 1988; Mahoney & Gabriel, 1987; Reda, 1986; Sroufe & Rutter, 1984).

2. The usual methodology is descriptive in the sense that def-

initions coincide with descriptions of clinical features of the disorders, and in this way seem to shape the attempt, old but still effective, to resolve a problem by omitting it. In fact, the problem lies precisely in rendering intelligible how and why the clinical features observed exhibit the characteristics that, descriptively, they do indeed possess (Weimer, 1982). Hence, it is doubtful what use, whether in clinical research or in psychotherapeutic practice, techniques of assessment may have when based on such a methodological program. In this respect, Faust and Miner (1986) point out: "if theories only summarize descriptions, they are virutally useless. A theory that does only this is more like a filing system which knows and can discover only what is already discovered and known" (p. 966).

Furthermore, this methodological attitude in the long run becomes misleading in that it reifies the descriptive diagnostic categories with which it classifies the range of clinical features observed to the point where these categories begin to look like clothes that a subject might wear, according to circumstances. Consider, for example, the diagnostic category labeled as depression: it would seem that once out of a depressive episode (like removing an article of clothing) the person returns to a mode of being which is quite different from that in which he or she felt helpless. It is known, however, that even in periods of complete well-being, these subjects exhibit, albeit with lower frequency and intensity, attitudes, modes of thought, and emotional reactions that are perfectly analogous to those present in the acute phase (Reda, 1984). Identical, or closely matching, patterns are also seen when one considers the trend of psychophysiological parameters that reveal the basic sensory-perceptive attitude of the subject (Reda, Arciero, & Blanco, 1986; Reda, Blanco, Guidano, & Mahoney, 1988). It is thus clear how a depressive episode, far from being something which strikes the person from without, like a fever or disease, is intrinsically bound up with his or her way of assimilating experience, of evaluating it and integrating it with past data—in a word, within the coherence of his or her personal meaning.

Finally, the epistemological premise can no longer be maintained on which the empiricist principles of parsimony and objective description rest, that is, the existence—independent from us—of an unequivocal external order in which a "sense of things" is objectively contained which can be known as such through unbiased observations. As far as we know at this stage, it is impossible to distinguish our perception of the world from our being in it, and this testifies decidedly against that external, unequivocal order which we have dreamed of and cherished since the time of Bacon (Jantsch, 1980; Maturana, 1988a; Maturana & Varela, 1987; Olafson, 1988; Varela, 1979, 1984). If knowledge cannot be a reasonably faithful copy of an order existing independently of it, we lose any possibility of evaluating it according to criteria of objectivity valid in themselves. So it would seem that the rationalist attitude of assuming the existence of standard logical axioms on the basis of which one may evaluate the rationality of any belief or attitude, independently of the whole functioning of the subject exhibiting it, is part and parcel of this same atheoretical and descriptive methodology.

A developmental approach to psychopathology centered on a systems/process-oriented methodology should instead lead us to the generation of a true science of personal meaning, that is, an approach that not only takes into account the multiplicity of levels of analysis within a complex individual unit, but is also able to reconstruct the whole array of reciprocal intercorrelations defining the coherence of the functioning of the whole. In this light, for example, it would no longer make much sense to talk of anxiety as a psychopathological category as such, and thus unequivocal for all. Anxiety as such (like other negative emotions of clinical interest) is part of a range of emotional tonalities with which humans experience their world. Within this same human experience, however, there exist different patterns of meaning coherence, so the same emotional tonality may be ordered and experienced in correspondingly different ways. Hence, a phobic coherence will scaffold anxiety in terms of protection/constriction, a depressive will do so in terms of losses, an eating disorders in terms of disappointments, and, finally, an obsessive in terms of lack of certainty.

Briefly, the methodological underpinnings of such a science of meaning revolve around the following points:

Each individual unit is to be considered as a Personal Meaning Organization (P.M.Org.) whose ontological understanding viably consists of "bringing-forth-a-world" capable of producing a quality of self-perception ("I") recognizable as one's own self ("Me"). Each P.M.Org. has its own self-referent ordering logic—as viable and coherent as that of any other—which allows it to assimilate experience in a manner consonant with its selfhood dynamics and the orthogenetic directionality deriving from it.

Lifespan development should be regarded as an open process of experience assimilation bringing about "punctuated" reorganizations of personal meaning. On the other hand, it is quite evident that no reorganization—not even if it brings about truly deep personal growth—is completely painless, as it always requires a change in the usual way of perceiving reality. This implies a triggering of intense feelings that appear, at least at first, to be neither readily intelligible nor easily controllable. Therefore, the P.M.Org.'s level of self-awareness (i.e., to what extent the "Me" viably recognizes the "I") exerts a crucial role in orienting an ongoing reorganization process toward a direction of personal growth or toward one of existential breakdown more or less intermingled with emotional disturbances. For this reason the "symptoms" an individual system may display at any stage of its lifespan must be considered as fully fledged knowing processes highlighting unsuccessful attempts to change, whose origin goes back to a poor or nonviable level of awareness that prevents a coherent assimilation of the personal experience produced thus far.

The essential tension inherent in selfhood dynamics underlies the progressive unfolding of personal meaning as well as its punctuated reorganizations, thereby constraining the generative directionality of any individual lifespan. As a consequence, the causes of a "crisis" are always within the P.M.Org. itself, and should therefore not be sought in a supposed specificity of certain stressful life events, but rather in the specific nature of personal meaning which determines the range of events that are discrepant for one particular individual. On the other hand, the critical role that a life event can play does not necessarily imply that such meaning needs to be consciously processed, since often what appears as a nonsense to the "Me" is in fact critical in the experiencing "I." The relatively autonomous emergence of critical feelings signaling an ongoing change in the "Me" appraisal of the "I" is made possible precisely by the proactive processes inherent in selfhood dynamics.

Mental Disorders and Dimensions of Systemic Coherence

As one might expect, an atheoretical and descriptive psychopathology has profoundly influenced even basic notions regarding mental health (i.e., normalcy) and mental disorders (i.e., neurosis and psychosis). In a nutshell, normalcy, neurosis, and psychosis have always been considered static, fixed *entities* which function as filing instruments for making an inventory of the descriptive features held to be specific. Considering knowledge as a copy of external order, assimilated in turn by a set of standard axioms (e.g., hedonistic motivation, logic procedures, etc.), it became possible, on the basis of the degree of correspondence to such a set, to define those descriptive features in terms of specific knowledge *contents* (beliefs, emotions, attitudes, etc.) identifying normal, neurotic, or psychotic behavior.

Now, the problem, as we know, is not so much that of evaluating how human beings keep to a presumed order independent of themselves, but rather that of understanding which experiencing of themselves accompanies their constructing the coherent order with which they coexist. Thus, rather than being identified with descriptive features of knowledge content, normalcy, neurosis, and psychosis are considered conceptual categories that refer to the organizations of personal meaning (P.M.Orgs.) which, making knowledge contents coherent, are causally productive of those features. On the other hand, the P.M.Orgs. outlined above should be considered as unitary ordering processes whose coherence and continuity can be grasped only in the specificity of the formal, structural properties of their knowledge processing, rather than in the definite semantic aspects of their knowledge contents. Hence, normalcy—which in accord with Levine (1949) we hold to be "non-existent in a complete form, but existing as relative and quantitative approximation"—rather than being an entity identified with something considered "normal" P.M.Org. or "normal" knowledge content, lies instead in the unfolding of a dynamic process, that is, the flexibility, resilience, and generativity with which a specific P.M.Org. develops its systemic coherence throughout lifespan, and in the higher levels of organized complexity and self-transcendence that it is consequently able to achieve. In the same way, "psychotic" refers to a structural modality of knowledge ordering whose coherence reduces flexibility and resilience; a delusional attitude, for example, is not thus because its thought content is not "close-to-reality," but rather because this thought content (which of itself is also present in normalcy) is more difficult to integrate with other contents, and thus less susceptible to being transformed by the current experience.

In a systems/process-oriented methodology, therefore, normalcy, neurosis, and psychosis—rather than being seen as descriptive and static entities—should be regarded as dynamic and changeable *processing dimensions* of a P.M.Org.'s systemic coherence, which appear to be potentially reversible, as their borders are indistinct most of the time (Marmor, 1983; Schwartz, 1987). Consequently, along the normalcy–psychosis continuum, normalcy corresponds to the flexibility and generativity with which a P.M.Org. articulates its fundamental orthogenetic directionality throughout lifespan. On the other hand, the *same* P.M.Org., depending on the quality and processing of developmental experiences, can evolve toward a "neurotic" dimension if the concreteness–abstractness level of knowledge processing is insufficiently articulated, or drift toward a "psychotic" dimension if, in addition to the limit represented by too concrete processing, there is also interference in the self-synthesizing integrative ability which provides functional unity to selfhood dynamics (Guidano, 1987). In other words, neurosis and psychosis are nothing but different "languages"—matched by correspondingly different dimensions of immediate experiencing and self-reflexive consciousness—that the same pattern of meaning coherence can assume as a function of the individual's processing and integrating abilities (Figure 1). The assumption that any pattern of meaning may be articulated along normal, neurotic, or psychotic dimensions permits us to better understand the nosographic categories that turn out to be confirmed (such as depression) and to lay down the basis for revising nosographic categories that seem uncertain (such as schizophrenia).

As far as depression is concerned, its appearance as a defined

DIMENSIONS OF SYSTEMIC COHERENCE		
NORMALCY	NEUROSIS	PSYCHOSIS
Flexibility	< Flexibility	<< Flexibility
Concreteness abstraction ——————→	Concreteness abstraction ←————	Concreteness abstraction ←————
Self-Integration ——————→	Self-Integration ——————→	Self-Integration ←————

FIGURE 1

nosographic category derives exclusively from the fact that the descriptive clinical features employed in its definition almost all belong to the same pattern of personal meaning (helplessness/anger oscillations). Now, it is precisely depression which can demonstrate how the same pattern of systemic coherence may be articulated along a continuum of processing dimensions. We need only think how the same experience of loss may be processed in a generative, creative way, giving rise to professional, artistic, or simply human sensitivity which is manifested in a high level of abstraction ("normal" dimension); or to an interrupted chain of losses and grief reactions as if one had to "concretely" face an inexorable destiny of exclusion ("neurotic" dimension); or, again, when transformations in the ordinary level of self-consciousness (i.e., "delusions" varying according to "negative" [helplessness] or "positive" [anger] mood oscillations) become the essential way of managing nonintegrable, too concrete experiences of loss or anger ("psychotic" dimension). It will be seen, finally, that such dimensions, being reversible and having rather indistinct borders, may overlap each other in a variety of ways along the same individual lifespan.

Regarding schizophrenia, however, the heterogeneity of descriptive clinical features used in the nosographic definitions has always impeded the formulation of a unitary, etiopathogenic hypothesis which is reliable, so much so that its role as a nosographic category in itself has even been called into question. This doubt becomes even more consistent if different clinical observations made by longitudinal studies in recent years are considered.

In the first place, a significant proportion of schizophrenics have only one episode from which they recover, and an even larger proportion show a course of several episodes before final remission. Only a small proportion reach chronicity, but evidence also shows that there is considerable doubt whether much of the chronicity is indigenous to schizophrenia; there is reason to believe that it may be an artifact engendered by iatrogenic, ecogenic, and nosocomial factors (Zubin, Steinhauer, Day, & van Kammen, 1985).

Secondly, various data show that a substantial continuity exists between the structure of personality reconstructible before the episode and that which is seen after remission. After remission, moreover, an emotional disorder of phobic, obsessive–compulsive, or other previously described types may appear, that is, a disorder not belonging in any way to the schizophrenic typology; this same disturbance existed in a more or less intense, but always reconstructible fashion, even *before* the appearance of the episode (Ballerini & Rossi Monti, 1983).

It would thus seem legitimate to suppose that when we use the term schizophrenia, we refer to the descriptive clinical features corresponding to acute, critical episodes of nonintegrated self-processing, episodes at which different patterns of personal meaning may arrive as a function of the quality of their ongoing "I"/"Me" dynamics. As we have seen, each P.M.Org. exhibits its own specific vulnerability in being able to reach critical points of self-integration, whether under the form of "wavering self" (eating disorders), "dichotomous self" (obsessive–compulsive), or "sensorial self" (phobic).

4

Self-Boundaries and
Lifespan Development

The key feature underlying the autonomy of any P.M.Org.
consists of the ability to transform into experience consistent with its
pattern of coherence (self-referent order) the randomness of perturbations coming both from the environment and from its own inner
oscillations (the so-called "order-from-noise" principle; Atlan, 1981,
1984). The lifespan development of a P.M.Org. should therefore be
regarded as an open-ended, spiraling process, in which the continuous
reordering of selfhood dynamics brings about the discontinuous emergence of more structured and integrated patterns of meaning coherence. The self-regulating ability exhibited by a P.M.Org. in proceeding along its orthogenetic directionality is expressed by that particular
dynamic equilibrium known as "order through fluctuations" (Brent,
1978; Dell & Goolishian, 1981; Prigogine, 1976); that is, continuous—both progressive and regressive—shifts of the point of equilibrium in "I"/"Me" dynamics are the only way of maintaining the
coherence that scaffolds the continuity of one's experiencing, while at
the same time assimilating the perturbations that emerge from that
experiencing. In order to give a clearer picture of such a process, it will
help if we first take a look at the essential variables that regulate its
dynamics: the role of awareness in regulating and modulating challenging
perturbations, and the role of affectivity in triggering them.

AWARENESS AND SELF-REGULATION

In the discussion of self-boundary development (Chapter 2), we
indicated that awareness relates to the abstract-reflexive dimension

65

through which immediate experiencing ("I") is self-referred in order to be consistently reordered into the self-image currently appraised ("Me). From adolescence on, reflexive self-referring gradually becomes an essential regulator and modulator of "I"/"Me" dynamics, so that any possible reorganization of self-boundary coherence during the subsequent lifespan is constrained by concomitant shifts in the unfolding of the abstract dimension of awareness. This is therefore a suitable place to consider briefly the essential aspects underlying the dynamics of such reflexive self-regulation before outlining the relationship between awareness and meaning coherence.

Awareness and Selfhood Dynamics

Basically, awareness regulates the essential tension inherent in selfhood dynamics, that is to say, the way in which the "Me" keeps up with (reordering itself) the acting and experiencing "I" which is always one step ahead of the current appraisal of the situation. Immediate experiencing is constantly matched by an automatic scaffolding of relevant information, which occurs independently from the selective attention intentionally carried out by the conscious self. More specifically, the level and quality of emotional modulation raised by automatic processes constrain the pathways of activation along which immediate processing proceeds (Hasher & Zacks, 1979, 1984; Posner & Snyder, 1975). While attending to ongoing events, the recurrent oscillation of the unitary network of nuclear scenes orders the flowing of psychophysiological rhythms into feeling tonalities and emotional experiences which are able to specify moment by moment the perceived quality of one's being-in-the-world. Indeed, because of the organizational unity of the emotional domain, the emotionality connected with automatic processing—via spreading activation—is invariably matched by the implicit ordering in terms of personal meaning, giving consistency and continuity in time to the immediate self experienced moment by moment (Collins & Loftus, 1975; Dixon, 1981; Van den Berg & Eelen, 1984). We are thus dealing with a specific apprehension of the world which tags incoming data with a feeling of self-reference from which the data immediately acquire a specific configuration in the subject's pre-existing personal experience. The activation of stored data, resulting from the attunement of past experiences with current ones, is a retrieval carried out by means of an analogue procedure, similar to that described by Tulving (1972, 1983, 1985) with the term "episodic memory" (i.e., an emotional memory mechanism which, through the retrieval of the perceptual features and feeling tonalities with which the memories were experienced, brings forth an immediate reference to one's perceived continuity). However, while the emotional modulation provided by the experiencing "I" can exceed a certain threshold as it slips in and out of the focus of consciousness, the effective possibilities of its being appraised and recognized as one's conscious self ("Me") depend on the abstract abilities of self-referring which have so far been structured.

Any explicit reordering is a self-referent procedure aimed at stabilizing the established patterns of immediate experience ("I") upon which the perceived coherence of the conscious self ("Me") depends. On the one hand, the ongoing tacit scaffolding constrains the set of experiences allowed to proceed to the conscious level, and on the other, the consistency of explicit reordering results, primarily, from perceiving this very set as stable and continuous in time. Thus, an immediate experience is made understandable through a selective appraisal of the sensory-affective-motor features already recognized as its own by the current self-image. Self-conscious processes, in turn, have an amplifying function on the perception of recognizable features, while at the same time inhibiting the detection of other cues (Cowan, 1988; Posner & Snyder, 1975; Spitzer, De Simone, & Moran, 1988). Therefore, any explication of immediate experiencing corresponds to a construction from the point of view of the "Me" that is carrying it out, and is consequently aimed at confirming the current appraisal of the world rather than at exploring the experiencing "I." Thus, the restructuring of episodic into *semantic memory* (Tulving, 1972, 1985) involves abstracting from a perceptual-emotional storage (e.g., the experience of anger) expectations and thought procedures to the perceived experience consistent with the sense of personal continuity (e.g., having cognitions about one's own experiencing of anger in keeping with the selected self-image).

More specifically, through the abstract self-referring that characterizes the "Me"-appraisal-of-the"I," the ongoing psychophysiological modulation is reordered into sequences of conscious emotional states, that is to say, into affective experiences able to support and further specify one's perceived uniqueness. The self-attribution of analogue/emotional processing is carried out through a set of specific semantic dimensions (Lang, 1984; Schwartz & Trabasso, 1984), which can be summarized as follows:

1. Valence, or polarity, accounts for a majority of the variance in affective reports and involves locating perceived feelings within the pleasure–displeasure continuum. As a basic and immediate distinguishable property of affective arousal, it concerns mainly an appraisal of the *intensity* with which the "Me" is affected by the experiencing "I," and is consequently reflected by oscillations in approach–avoidance dispositions.
2. The pattern and the directness of the arousal, as a further elaboration, affect the appraisal of the *quality* of the experienced affect, allowing a discrimination of the emotional content (i.e., imagery/memory modulation) as well as a patterning of psychophysiological responses (i.e., bodily sensations and motor activity).
3. As a final step, the self–other reference distinction specifies whether the experienced affect is perceived as "internally bound" and recognized as belonging to one's own self, or as "externally bound" and attributed to other causes than the self, such as the environment or the body itself. In general, internal reference brings about a control of emotion through understanding, thus facilitating further articulations in abstract self-referring. External attribution, however, gives rise to control of emotions based on their exclusion, and is matched by a sense of being at the mercy of unpredictable events and impulses which adversely affects self-analytical abilities.

It is relevant to notice how cues for decoding valence and directedness derive directly from the emotional modulation carried out by the experiencing "I," while cues for self–other reference mainly derive from the patterns of coherence enacted by the "Me." Given that immediate experience and its conscious appraisal are matched by different dimensions of knowing processes (i.e., ordering and reordering levels), feelings can exist in consciousness independently of cognition (Izard, 1977; Zajonc, 1984; Zajonc & Markus, 1984). In the absence of cognitive decoding, however, their motor and autonomic activation tends to be directly realized through somatic or motor manifestations of emotion. These are likely to be experienced as fairly uncontrollable floating states overflowing one's usual range of recognizable emotions. As a consequence, an experienced affect will be perceived as an externally bound perturbation to the extent to which it does not fit with the range of decodability allowed by current patterns of coherence.

Therefore, as a multilevel and mulidirectional process, continuous self-reordering is inherently characterized, moment by moment, by a series of possible *"I"/"Me" discrepancies*, that is, perceived gaps between immediate experience and self-consciousness that challenge ongoing patterns of self-control. The perturbing experience of overflowing one's usual range of recognizable emotions is generally kept within acceptable limits by a dynamic equilibrium in which conscious attention selectively amplifies the current self-image, while at the same time inhibiting potential discrepancies from rising into active awareness. As studies on self-encoding processes have by now shown, when reordering immediate experience, people have virtually unlimited access to past and current data they intend to look for, and people themselves set the limits of the research (Bower & Gilligan, 1979; Gilligan & Bower, 1984; Mancuso & Ceely, 1980; Markus, 1977).

Awareness and Meaning Coherence

In strictly ontological terms, being aware of oneself means reaching an explanation for the ongoing experience of being a unique, irreducible and, often, unpredictable "I." As Nagel (1979) has pointed out: "an organism has conscious mental states if and only if there is something that it is like to *be* that organism—something it is like *for* the organism" (p. 166). This means that immediate experiencing is the "given" epistemic level that constrains any attempt at self-explanation and on which any attained self-explanation depends. Gadamer (1979) highlights this clearly and elegantly:

> Long before we understand ourselves through the process of self-examination, we understand ourselves in a self-evident way in the family, society and state in which we live. The focus of subjectivity is a distorting mirror. The self-awareness of the individual is only a flickering in the closed circuits of historical life. That is why prejudices of the individual, far more than his judgements, constitute the historical reality of his being. (p. 245)

Hence, more than being an image of oneself objectively seen from outside, awareness is a reflexive process for self-referring immediate experience ("I") which, through a continuous allocation of attention and intention, aims at amplifying consistent aspects of the perceived "Me," while inhibiting discrepant ones. Little wonder, then, if from the external point of view of an "objective reality," verbal reports appear unreliable as *valid* descriptions of people's immediate experience (see Nisbett & Wilson, 1977). As a matter of fact, their function is to provide explanations of one's experiencing *viable* for the internal viewpoint of one's sense of continuity. Therefore, rather than more or less reliable "snapshots" of internal states, conscious self-reports should be regarded as procedures for making them consistent with the current self-image, on the basis both of the specific pattern of internal coherence and of the level of abstractness and flexibility with which it is carried out (Ketterer, 1985; Miller, 1981; White, 1980, 1988).

Furthermore, the essential tension inherent in selfhood dynamics, allowing one to experience more than one perceives and to perceive more than one attends to, makes it possible that in any situation we are all in a position to experience much more than that which would be required at that moment to maintain our own consistency in that situation. As a consequence, the ability to manipulate immediate experiencing while self-referring and reordering it becomes essential, done in such a way as to impede the arising into consciousness of irrelevant data, or of data that contrast with the selected appraisal of the situation currently underway. Finally, if we consider how, from its very first emergence, reflexive self-referring entails the capacity for conscious deception, it will be seen that no self-awareness will be viable without adequate self-deception. Excessive self-deception raises the undecodability of immediate experiencing to critical levels of uncontrollability, while reduced self-deception increases self-referring processes out of all proportion, easily reaching levels of complexity in selfhood dynamics which would be difficult to manage. Hence, any P.M.Org., while being characterized by critical emotive tonalities in immediate experiencing, is also endowed with specific self-deceiving procedures designed to manipulate their decoding so it is consistent with the quality of awareness allowed by its level of abstractness and flexibility. Through such procedures, critical feelings can be appraised and made intelligible without calling into question the self-image acceptability so far structured (see Chapter 3, "I"/"Me" dynamics in P.M.Orgs.).

Moreover, in the dynamic equilibrium between the ongoingness of immediate experiencing and current patterns of awareness, the regulating role played by self-deceiving procedures is twofold: while aiming at preserving the current equilibrium, they also, at the same time, create the conditions for the emergence of "I"/"Me" discrepancies, assimilation of which entails shifts of the point of equilibrium in the direction of either a progressive or regressive personal reordering, according to the level of abstractness and flexibility of awareness. In regressive reorderings, the challenging of current self-control is always matched by remarkable levels of overemotionality and personal imbalance which often take on all the characteristics of cognitive dysfunctions and emotional disorders usually exhibited by clinical syndromes; the greater the undecodability of the "I"/"Me" discrepancy emerging, the more intense will be the "splitting" experienced between one's thoughts and feelings (Guidano, 1987). On the one hand, conscious explicit processing will be more and more focused to maintain to the utmost the current self-image through the elaboration of cognitions and behavior that deny the discrepant feelings, which come to be perceived as something extraneous to the self. On the other hand, lacking a proper cognitive mediation, the motor, autonomic, and affective setting that accompanies the ongoing activation of discrepant, uncontrollable feelings tends to be directly actualized; the activation meets no delays on the road to its terminus: emotional outbursts, somatic disturbances, and stereotyped behavior.

LOVE AND AFFECTIVE STYLE
AS ATTACHMENT PROCESSES

As the "cognitive revolution" takes place in adolescence and youth, attachment, although shifting toward a more abstract level, maintains its fundamental interdependence with selfhood dynamics and personal meaning. While attachment to significant others is central to the differentiation of self-boundaries throughout maturational stages, during adulthood, new patterns of attachment emerge (e.g., intimate love relationships) which acquire the self-referent function of confirming, supporting, and further expanding the pattern of personal meaning coherence which has so far been structured. It follows naturally that the influence of early attachments is now seen in the style of attachment, which, having begun in early models, has continued to differentiate along the entire developmental pathway (Bretherton, 1985).

Disregarding for the moment the different forms that it can take, the continuity of attachment during lifespan is understandable if we consider that the involvement with affective relationships perceived as unique begins early in life, and adult bonds of love seem to grow out of those very first attachments (Hazan & Shaver, 1987; Marris, 1982; Shaver, Hazan, & Bradshaw, 1988; Weiss, 1982). Just as the uniqueness of primary bonds seems to be a necessary requisite for perceiving-a-world and recognizing one's being-in-it, so in adulthood, even though at a different level of abstraction, building a unique relationship with a significant other is an important way in which one may perceive a consistent sense of uniqueness in his or her being-in-the-world. Hence, if working models of attachment figures are interdependent with ongoing patterns of self-perception, it is clear that any perceived modification of these models is matched by intense perturbations in immediate experiencing; these perturbations can trigger the emergence of "I"/"Me" discrepancies, which in turn challenge the current appraisal of the self. In point of fact, the importance of a balanced interplay of the individual's network of unique relationships during lifespan is currently supported by evidence from various sources. Firstly, life-events research has shown that the most disrupting emotions a person can ever experience in life are those triggered in the course of establishing, maintaining, and breaking such relationships (Bowlby, 1977; Brown, 1982; Hafner, 1986; Henderson, 1982; Henderson, Byrne, & Duncan-Jones, 1981). Secondly, recent epidemiological evidence has shown how the "social network index" should be regarded as a significant predictor of health, since social and affective isolation is a major risk factor for morbidity and mortality (House, Landis, & Umberson, 1988).

These data make the intersubjective nature of human experience even more evident, and therefore a closer analysis of the interdependence between attachment and selfhood processes is warranted.

Attachment, Perceived Uniqueness,
and Selfhood Dynamics

The intersubjectivity inherent in attachment systems unfolds through a basic self-referent process articulated along different levels of abstraction and processing abilities according to the developmental phases of the individual lifespan. Thus, in the earliest periods the internalization of an attachment figure through emotional identification is matched by an intermodal patterning of sensory-motor-affective modules into a unitary configuration which brings forth a specific sense of self and the world. In the same way, the more abstract construction of attachment figures resulting from adult love relationships is paralleled by a reordering of immediate experience that is perceived in a variety of ways according to the specific selfhood dynamics inherent in the individual. In this sense, adult bonding corresponds to the scaffolding of a synchrony between psychophysiological rhythms of both members of the pair, matched by a behavioral meshing of their interactional patterns (Field, 1985; Field & Reite, 1985; Hinde, 1979; Kelley et al., 1983). Through the selective emotional modulation that they can provide, intersubjective reciprocal attunements work as basic regulators of selfhood dynamics, allowing the "Me" to recognize the perceived uniqueness of the experienced "I" as consistent in time. This regulatory role, together with the sensory, motor, and temporal patterning of actual interactions, also includes the whole stream of significant interpersonal experiences, and, therefore, past close relationships. Attributes extracted from past attachment figures trigger memories intermingled with expectancies that involve the activation of sensory-motor-affective patterns, thus bringing about specific qualities of self-perception.

Hence, as Hofer (1984) notes, independent self-regulation does not exist in adulthood or in childhood, and intersubjectivity is constrained by a basic self-referent ordering through which the construction of a significant other's image comes to be correlated to a perception of self. On the other hand, only by considering the image of the other, not so much as a mere "cognitive representation," but rather as an intermodal coordination of sensory-motor-affective modules, does it become understandable how the presence of, or physical contact with, another person can modulate human cardiovascular activity and reactivity in general and, particularly, in stressful situations (House, Landis, & Umberson, 1988; Melnechuk, 1988; Panksepp, Siviy, & Normansell, 1985).

In other words, assuming a systems/process-oriented methodology, attachment can no longer be considered a mere structural device for the maintaining of proximity and contact with a significant figure, as is usually the case in descriptive methodologies based on empiricist principles of parsimony (Trevarthen, 1980, 1984). Within an ontological perspective trying to explain how a human being comes to experience a unique and specific sense of individuality, attachment becomes the self-referential system that preeminently underlies the development and maintenance of selfhood dynamics. That is, the unfolding ability to take others' perspectives on oneself is paralleled by the progressive ability to reorder immediate experience ("I") in such a way as to make it recognizable and understandable in terms of one's own self ("Me").

Furthermore, within the intersubjective dimension inherent in human experience, the perceived uniqueness of one's being-a-person lies in the dynamic intersection of a multilevel and oscillative process. No human being can perceive a sense of self independently of empathic attunement with significant others' consciousness of him- or herself; at the same time, this sense of self results from an active differentiation between one's felt subjectivity and the perceived objectivity of others' perspective.

> . . . the unity of the person, which is constructed by way of intersubjectively recognized self-identification (analyzed by G. H. Mead) is based on belonging to, and demarcating oneself from, the symbolic reality of a group, and on the possibility of locating oneself in it. (Habermas, 1979, p. 109)

Finally, during lifespan development, the unfolding of the opponent regulative dynamics between "belonging to" and "demarcating from" takes on the form of an endless process of negotiating mutual consensus and acceptance; that is, at any moment, people engaged in an interpersonal context must act in such a way as to enable the differentiating-oneself-from-others to be recognized by those others. Gadamer emphasizes this aspect with accustomed lucidity, pointing out that

> the inner historicality of all the relations in the lives of men consists in the fact that there is a constant struggle for mutual recognition. This can have very varied degrees of tension, to the point of the complete domination of one person by the other; but even the most extreme forms of mastery and slavery are a genuine dialectical relationship. (1979, p. 323)

Bonding and Separation in Adulthood

In an ontological perspective, therefore, the crucial feature of an affective, close relationship reciprocally consists of a self-referent construction of an image of the significant other which can stabilize and, if need be, further develop the selfhood dynamics thus far structured. More specifically, the physiological linkage with the other's rhythms brings about a quality of immediate experiencing ("I") more specifically perceived as one's "real" self ("Me"). Thus, the course of a relationship is more closely linked to perceptions of the other than to actual characteristics of the other (Sternber & Barnes, 1985), so that in the process of bonding to somebody, one does not choose a person so much as the mode of experiencing oneself with that person. Let us briefly look at the essential variables which regulate a complex and dynamic process of this nature.

First of all, the quality of the other's constructed image is closely correlated to the pattern of personal meaning. Hence, in a depressive meaning, the other's image is always correlated to the sense of loneliness and exclusion from the interpersonal world either in a positive (redemption from a destiny of loneliness) or negative (confirmation of such a destiny) way. In phobic meaning, the need to be relieved from the fear of living in a dangerous world constrains any possible perception of an attachment figure, with the possibility of triggering a positive (protection without any perceived limit to one's need for freedom) or negative (perceived threats of losing protection and/or freedom and independence) immediate experiencing. In eating disorders, the image of an affective partner is perceived in terms of one's own consciousness, giving rise to the possibility of decreasing (the other's approvals perceived as absolutely noncontingent) or increasing (the other's perception as intruding and/or disconfirming) one's blurred and wavering immediate experience. And lastly, in the obsessive dimension, the need to unify and stabilize a dichotomous experiencing into a certain identity brings about two opposite possibilities that shift from one to the other in an "all-or-nothing" way; that is, either the perceived other confirms the certainty of having total control, or he or she is perceived as the only possibility for relieving one's distressing sense of uncontrollability.

Secondly, the development of the immediate experience, derived from the type of image that has been constructed, depends on the *degree* and *quality* of emotional reciprocity in the affective relationship.

As far as the *degree* is concerned, it is now clear that the perceived closeness of an attachment figure is highly correlated to the intensity of emotional interdependence experienced in the relationship (Berscheid, 1983; Berscheid, Gangestad, & Kulakowski, 1984; Kelley et al., 1983). Thus, the degree of closeness becomes a good predictor of emotional reactions if the relationship dissolves, and here also is a clue for understanding how even intensely negative relationships produce a level of physiological linkage and interrelatedness that can trigger intense grief reactions during the process of separation (Clark & Reis, 1988; Levenson & Gottman, 1983).

The *quality* of emotive reciprocity depends on the type of negotiation for mutual recognition which has been set up in the relationship.

From one point of view, in order to realize the possibility of an effective negotiation, the partner must in some way be perceived in one's own "range," so that negative emotions are invariably triggered if the perceived esteem for the partner is either too high or too low (Tesser, 1987). As was noted more than three centuries ago by La Rochefoucauld (1678/1959), "it is difficult to love people that we do not esteem, but it is no less difficult to love those whom we esteem much more than ourselves." From another point of view, the critical variable is the type of response perceived in the opposite party to one's affective style, which is to say, to the set of strategies marshaled to obtain recognition and confirmation of one's selfhood dynamics.

To each pattern of personal meaning there corresponds, moreover, a specific affective style. Thus, a depressive style will try to obtain an unconditional acceptance of one's perceived unlovableness through the rhythmic oscillation between emotional detachment and compulsive caregiving. An eating disorders style will seek a supportive intimacy that demands minimal self-exposure through a whole repertoire of "tests and retests" for the partner. Lastly, a style centered on an effective control over all aspects of the relationship will be the preferred strategy both in phobic (where overcontrolling the partner supplies the indispensable "protective" base while confirming one's need for freedom) and in obsessive style (where being in the "one-up" role coincides with proposing oneself as the indisputable holder of absolute certainties and truths).

It is clear that, within a continually tranforming long-lasting relationship, each of these styles is able to produce a wide range of both recognitions and disconfirmations of one's selfhood dynamics. We do feel, however, that it is important to emphasize how a specific affective style is able to produce, in the same relationship, both an emotional reciprocity experientiable as a secure attachment, and a reciprocal conflictuality confirming the supposed impossibility of attaining the desired security. In other words, in the lifespan unfolding of personal meaning, an attachment style functions as a "boundary-maintaining system" which is able to produce in any phase of an ongoing relationship a quality of immediate experience in keeping with the continuity of one's perceived coherence.

In considering relationship dissolution, we shall distinguish, for simplicity's sake, two aspects which are in reality closely intertwined and so somewhat indistinguishable: the nature and dynamics of separation and the distressing emotional reaction (grieving) connected with it.

Regarding the nature of separation, it is important to note that, as with any other lifespan structure, affective ties follow an orthogenetic directionality progressively differentiating through developmental changes from a state of undifferentiated globality to more integrated levels of structural order and hierarchical organization. As we would intuitively expect, the initial dimension of a relationship is relatively global and undifferentiated, insofar as it coincides with the immediate aspects of the emotional involvement (attraction, self-disclosure, sexual agreement/harmony/caring, etc.) which plays a role in the reciprocal selection. As the relationship proceeds, however, these same aspects, giving rise to a new intersubjective context (marriage, childbirth, choices in career and work, reorganization of the social network, etc.), develop into more articulated dimensions of emotional interdependence (intimacy, reciprocal commitment, etc.) that acquire more and more the function of validating the sense of self of each dyad member.

Hence, relationship development progressively becomes a multilevel and multidirectional process, in which emergent dimensions of exchanges, acquiring their own orthogenetic course, will operate at different levels of the same relationship, requiring for their functioning a continuous process of hierarchical integration. Given that progress in hierarchical organization is seldom smooth, flexibility in integrating emergent emotional dimensions and new attribute domains is matched by oscillations in the quality of emotional interdependence (ups and downs in perceived involvement) as well as variability in reciprocal attitudes (shifting between affection and hostility). These recurrent oscillations in themselves do not reveal regressive aspects foreboding dissolution, in that they are simply phenomenal indicators of the continuous reordering taking place within a complex and changing system such as an affective relationship (Lerner, 1984). More specifically, it is the presence of minimal (low flexibility) or maximal (high instability) oscillations that positively correlates to the termination of a relationship.

> A relationship might survive one or even a few minimally or maximally oscillating dimensions—especially at early levels of relationship development, when fewer dimensions exist and when they are relatively more global (i.e., behaviorally more stereotyped) and hence less variable; but no relationship could be expected to survive when most dimensions, especially key ones, exhibit relatively minimal or maximal variability. If this should happen, the relationship would dissolve and, in a sense, return to a state analogous to its initial one. It will exist in a global state of no-longer-existing. In a sense, all relationships develop towards this end, as when the death of a dyad member occurs. (Lerner, 1984, p. 133)

The notion that relationships do not have endless duration and the probabilities of dissolution are "internal" (i.e., directly correlated to the flexibility with which a dyad reorders its own experience) gives us a better appreciation of the dynamics of separation.

First of all, it is clear that the reasons for the break-up of a relationship are not so much due to the supposed specificity of particular life events as to the dyad's available capacity for integrating challenging perturbations into generative dimensions. The development of a conjugal crisis will thus be even more unpredictable if evaluated solely as a function of the event that triggered it, given that a major unbalance may lead both to an irreversible breakdown and to a greater involvement in the generation of new commitments.

Secondly, rather than considering separation as merely a more or less distressing *event*, it should be regarded as a complex and multidirectional *process* that unfolds and takes on form through time (Duck, 1982; Lee, 1984). More specifically, the unfolding of an oscillatory process between approach and avoidance patterns, whose recurrence becomes more and more repetitive and stereotyped, seems to be characteristic of any affective separation, so it is found both in the termination stage of adult love relationships (Baxter, 1984) and in the course of the "physiological" adolescent–parental separation (Bloom, 1980). The intensity and duration of such an oscillatory process is directly correlated to the degree of emotional interdependence structured so far, to the point where one not infrequently observes that in many close relationships the process of separation ends up becoming the quantitatively most important phase of the whole relationship.

The duration of the separation process is related to the extent of the distressing grief that accompanies it. The term "grief" refers to the psychophysiological processes triggered by the experience of privation of a loved person, processes which reveal a reciprocal interconnection between the perception of loss and feelings of helplessness, sadness, and anger. Widespread among human and nonhuman primates (Rosenblum & Paully, 1987; Suomi, 1984), this interconnection rests on genetically wired apprehensional schemata in which loss represents the adaptive knowing dimension for scaffolding basic feelings (helplessness, anger, etc.) into specific emotional modulations which, increasing group cohesion, become viable for survival. This is not the place for an in-depth discussion of the data available on bereavement and grieving; however, it is evident from them that grieving is a process that unfolds in time through a sequence of stages (e.g., roughly, accepting and experiencing loss and, subsequently, reordering one's self-image in order to reinvest in other relationships; Bowlby, 1980; Parkes, 1972, 1982; Parkes & Weiss, 1983; Worden, 1982; Zisook, 1988). I shall confine myself to some considerations which will allow the further development of the ontological perspective which has been carried forward to this point.

If in bonding one chooses not so much the person as the way of experiencing oneself in relating to him or her, so in grieving what is experienced as lost is just this specific way of feeling rather than the "objective" absence of the person.

Given that the constructed image of an attachment figure regulates ongoing patterns of self-perception through intermodal coordinations of sensory-motor-affective modules, the crucial variable underlying any experience of being deprived of a loved one seems to be a rather abrupt change perceived in this image. Grieving, in turn, corresponds to a specific "I"/"Me" discrepancy, in which the experienced interruption of one's ongoing sense of self is matched by a distressing psychophysiological modulation. Evidence of the internal desynchronization and deregulation of psychophysiological rhythms in experiencing the interruption of a significant relationship supports the notion that the withdrawal of a previous regulation supplied by the attachment figure is at the base of the perceived alteration in established patterns of self-perception (Hofer, 1984; McGuire & Troisi, 1987). Moreover, if the "I"/"Me" discrepancy that results from grieving is centered on the perceived disintegration of one's continuity, it will be seen that subsequent attempts to restore continuity progressively lead to a complex process of personal reorganization which may develop progressively or regressively.

As the desynchronization between the image of the other and self-boundary regulation is at the core of both the experience of bereavement and the process of separation, there is a substantial continuity between the different grief reactions, no matter whether triggered by physical or affective losses. These two situations are nonetheless profoundly different as to the structure of the perceived change in the attachment figure: with death one loses physical and emotional contact but preserves the positivized image intact; in the case of an affective failure, it is precisely the image of the other that changes radically, usually negatively, while physical and emotional contact is usually maintained, owing to a variety of circumstances (children, work, common social network, etc.). The impression that one has from this, at least at a psychotherapeutic level, is that the loss of the image of the other without loss of contact is able to trigger grieving tonalities, less acute than bereavement, but far more ambiguous and ambivalent and which need more time to be completely processed and assimilated. The need to recover a "valuable" social role as soon as possible after a marriage dissolution, combined with the preceding difficulties in decoding immediate experience, all go to favor the establishment of grieving processes which are much more varied, or anomalous, than those met with in true mourning. Hence, the lesser emotional intensity when compared with bereavement favors the appearance of chronic grief reactions, as in those cases, for example, where the depressive state and social isolation following a divorce never come to a satisfactory conclusion. Under other circumstances, the emotional reaction is minimal during the process of separation and the grief appears to be delayed or postponed, with the tendency for recent losses, even minimal, to reactivate grieving for a loss sustained earlier (Bowlby, 1980). Lastly, people sometimes do not even minimally recognize that the difficulties being experienced are related to the loss that has occurred, and the grief reactions are masked as a result, and may thus take on the most diverse forms, ranging from clear-cut clinical disorders (e.g., phobic, obsessive imbalances) to maladaptive psychosomatic reactivity.

In light of these considerations, it should be clear that the

essential procedure underlying any attempt to avoid grieving by negat-
ing the loss involves the struggle to keep intact the image of the other
which has been structured up to this point. Basically, this procedure
works as a self-referent process in which the perceived unchangeability
of the other's image allows the subject to maintain his or her own
self-image. However, even though this is not in itself an anomalous
process, the difficulty of modifying the partner's image plays a significant role both in the process of separation and in the grieving that sets
in after the separation. Regarding the separation process, the continual oscillations between approach and avoidance would seem to reflect
such a difficulty, as if there had been a change of mind immediately
after perceiving the other as different from what one had thought.
Furthermore, it seems equally clear that these same stereotyped oscillations progressively and reciprocally erode the reliability perceived in
the other's image, thus making the progressive emotional detachment
irreversible.

Once the separation has taken place, however, the lower emotional intensity in comparison with true bereavement, together with
the compelling need to recover a consistent social role, concur to
divert attention from further processing of the grief experience, so that
both the other's image and one's own sense of self relating to him or
her are scarcely modified. In this way, the unfolding of anomalous
grief reactions appears to be closely correlated to the presence of
affective-memory mechanisms focused on the immediate experiences
which occurred in the relationship, on its dissolution, and on subsequent meetings. As Harvey, Flanary, and Morgan (1986) showed, the
more depressed people were after a separation, the more vivid and
"flashbulb-like" their memories were, suggesting that relating to the
partner was still intensely charged with emotions.

Consequently, reorganizing one's sense of continuity following a
separation depends, to a large extent, on the flexibility and generativity with which the subject is able to change the appraisal of the
relationship, as well as the emotional reciprocity enacted in it. In
proportion to the delay and/or reduction in such transformations,
anomalous grief reactions tend to persist indefinitely in time, becoming the habitual ingredients of immediate experience and giving rise to
maladaptive emotional attitudes, for example, perceived inability to
reinvest in other affective relationships, provocative behavior appear-
ing as soon as positive engagement is established, compulsive searching for impossible partners.

ADULTHOOD AND MEANING COHERENCE

The empiricist outlook regards the trend of an individual life-span after maturational stages as a sort of "plateau," as if adulthood consisted virtually of nothing more than maintaining indefinitely the optimal equilibrium that is thought to be attained by the end of the maturational period. This homeostatic perspective excludes any generative progression in lifespan, reducing adult development to a passive and cumulative process of data remodeling, regulated in any moment by contingency relationships established with the environment. If adulthood is a cumulation deprived of any generative role, then infancy, being at the very beginning of the cumulative process, logically becomes the only determining period of the entire life cycle. This assumption of the primacy of early years is tacitly or explicitly endorsed by most contemporary Western psychologies.

Rather than an "end product" or an "uninterrupted state," however, adulthood is an open-ended process of experience assimilation continuously shifting—either progressively or regressively—the attained point of equilibrium along the orthogenetic directionality of increasing its structural order and complexity (Baltes, 1979; Brent, 1978, 1984; Lerner & Busch-Rossnagel, 1981; Werner, 1957). Important changes in immediate experiencing and meaning coherence follow one upon the other throughout adulthood and aging, as the ever-growing array of nuclear scripts is continually transformed by new experiences so new levels of abstract self-referring matched by consequent new articulations in selfhood dynamics can be attained. Therefore, no specific moment of a lifespan can be identified as the one in which an ultimate, exhaustive understanding is achieved, nor is there any indication, within the individual's orthogenetic directionality, of the existence of a "right" or "optimal" equilibrium, or indeed of anything suggesting that an ultimate stage of maturity has been reached. As Gadamer (1979) puts it: "To exist historically means that knowledge of oneself can never be complete" (p. 269).

On the other hand, the orthogenetic progression, through which higher levels of internal complexity are attained while preserving one's sameness, implies that any developmental change involves a reordering of processes triggering discontinuity (the emergence of "I"/"Me" discrepancies) by processes preposed to restore continuity (self-awareness integrative abilities). Thus, any lifespan directionality unfolds through an essential tension between constancy and mutability, so that any developmental transformation always coincides with the emergence of a new dynamic equilibrium between the processes of maintenance and change.

Let us therefore briefly look at how the issues of continuity and change interplay and overlap within the main dimensions that regulate meaning coherence throughout adulthood.

Orthogenetic Directionality and Core Affective Themes

The unfolding of meaning coherence during lifespan development relies on the organizational unity of the individual's emotional domain. On the one hand, the rhythmic oscillation between core affective polarities scaffolds immediate experiencing along the same, continuous apprehensional dimensions; on the other, the endless process of self-referring and reordering the perceived continuity of immediate experience provides focus and direction in organizing thoughts, emotions, and actions along dimensions of self-awareness compatible with available levels of abstract processing.

Thus, the core affective theme maintains its prominence and continuity in the ideational themes (beliefs, philosophical axioms, self-conceptions, etc.) which follow one another during the whole course of adult life (Haviland, 1984; Malatesta & Clayton Culver, 1984; Stewart & Healy, 1984). However, ideational themes undergo a continuous process of change involving abstract differentiation and integration regulated by logical rules of transformation, while affective themes appear much more constant in time and seem to be pretty much unaffected by logical procedures in their rate and mechanism of change. In the first place, the articulation of affective themes from childhood and adolescent thematic contents takes place through an increasing number of relevant scenes made consistent through analogical rules of derivation and metaphorical projection whose spatiotemporal unfolding differs from the sequential linearity exhibited by thought processes. Secondly, any change in the affective theme is a result of the emergence of new emotional experiences which facilitate further articulations and transformations of immediate experiencing by adding new feeling tonalities and image schemata to the unitary configuration of core affective polarities.

Thus the basic procedure underlying lifespan directionality

seems to be the process of making the tacit explicit, whereby the ongoingness of immediate experiencing is constructively self-referred along the dimensions of semantic understanding (Guidano, 1987). Since the assimilation of emergent emotional tonalities facilitates the further articulation of immediate experiencing, the process of making the tacit explicit entails the structuring of self-maintained positive feedback leading to levels of even more complex and integrated symbolic-abstract processing. Consequently, the systemic coherence relating to each specific P.M.Org. constrains a preferential direction to its orthogenetic progression, in which the ascending toward higher abstract levels is matched by a progressive disengagement from the immediacy of one's experiencing of self. It is thus possible to broadly trace what might be the normative positive progression (i.e., that which coincides with a truly personal growth) for each of the P.M.Orgs. described in the previous chapter.

For a depressive meaning, the progressive directionality should be identified with a continuous differentiation and integration of the loss theme, until it is perceived as a category of human experience rather than as a personal destiny of loneliness and misery; the normative progression of eating disorder organization should lead to an ever-growing sense of one's uniqueness and individuality based on "internal criteria" rather than deriving it from the perceived attitudes of significant others; finally, in both phobic and obsessive meanings, the positive progression should lead (by way of totally different patterns and processes) to a growing sense of one's personal worth based on the progressive acknowledgment and appreciation of one's emotional domain and, consequently, to an increased ability to experience and understand, with minimal distress, the complexity and ambiguity inherent in the human interpersonal domain.

Needless to say, these directionalities represent "ideal" trajectories of adulthood that may be subject, at any time, to distortions and regressive shifts, and are always extremely variable from one person to another. They should therefore be regarded in the same way as one would identify an ideal or normative progression in maturational stages despite the wide range of normal or pathogenic developmental pathways that it can generate.

Reorganization of Meaning Coherence

The lifespan orthogenetic progression of any P.M.Org. does not have a linear course; quite the contrary, it is a somewhat unpredictable process that unfolds through critical, discontinuous emergings. Because of such critical increases in internal complexity, a P.M.Org. maintains its continuity only by shifting the current pattern of coherence toward a further articulation that implies a more or less thorough reorganization of its experiential order. Unlike maturational stages, the course of which is more linear and uniform, development in adulthood proceeds by crises that, in a sense, are reminiscent in many aspects of the pattern of "punctuated equilibria" proposed by post-Darwinian evolutionary approaches (see Gould, 1980; Lerner, 1984). Periods of stability in which the system seems to be only concerned with the maintenance of its status quo, thus becoming extremely predictable, are followed by very intense meta-stable periods in which the slightest perturbation unexpectedly triggers major existential crises and deep reorganization of personal experience (Allen, 1981; Brent, 1984).

On the other hand, the orthogenetic progression of an ontological system unfolds within an irreversible temporal direction. While we experience the irreversible direction of time from the past into the future as the "objective" temporal dimension, each of us experiences this irreversibility within a "subjective" time, flowing parallel to and perceived as interwoven with the objective temporal order. Moreover, any lifespan development is matched by the gradual emergence of changes in the subjective experience of time irreversibility, which becomes understandable in the light of the notion of "symmetry-breaking" processes introduced by Prigogine (1973), that is, as a history of progressive and irreversible differentiations between one's sense of past and future.

Each lifespan starts out with a virtually total temporal symmetry (i.e., the exclusive sense of the present that parallels, during infancy and childhood, the immediacy of the experiencing of self and reality). With the abstract self-referring that emerges during adolescence, this symmetry breaks down, bringing about a growing experiential differentiation between past and future. As one progresses in the lifespan, the experienced irreversibility of time directedness is projected into abstract reordering processes triggering transformations, equally irreversible, in one's sense of continuity. Thus, at the time of the "existential" discovery of the self in youth, the past is perceived as being just begun, and the person feels he or she faces an unlimited future full of potentialities. As time goes by, this sense of the future is replaced by another more restricted one, connected to the emerging awareness of death that takes place in early adulthood. With the beginning of middle age, the perceived finiteness of one's future progressively gives rise to the disturbing experience of being embodied, with no chance of escape, in a limited, unrepeatable and irreversible existence. Finally, in the course of aging, the future is less and less perceived as a projection toward alternative posibilities, and the sense of one's life is primarily based on a past that occupies, by now, nearly all of one's lifespan.

Needless to say, any transformation in the subjective perception of time is matched by a new space–time dimension that triggers a substantial reorganization of personal experience; any reorganization, in turn, exerts a great influence on the oscillations and transformations of the subsequent lifespan. It would therefore seem reasonable to hypothesize that the surfacing of symmetry-breaking processes roughly coincides with the gradual emergence of the critical periods of adulthood (e.g., adolescence, age-30 transition, midlife transition) which show up in longitudinal studies on life histories and biographies (Gould, 1978; Levinson, 1978, 1986; Sheehy, 1976; Stewart & Healy, 1984; Vaillant, 1977). However, compared to the greater uniformity in time and explanatory continuity of maturational critical periods, adult stages exhibit, even with the same character of invariant progression, greater variability and indeterminacy.

In the first place, individual differences in the concreteness–abstractness dimension strongly influence whether the appraisal of the emerging transformation in subjective time is made in terms of personal emotional domains or in terms of overwhelming experiences extraneous to the self. Secondly, individual differences in self-awareness deeply influence the quality of reorganization triggered by the critical period, and therefore the very structure of the final state attained. In other words, the continuity exhibited by maturational stages in which the orthogenetic progression is rigidly regulated by biological factors (unfolding of cognitive abilities), and so producing the same characteristics in the majority of subjects, is replaced in adult development by a greater indeterminacy, as orthogenetic progression now becomes regulated mainly by psychological factors (qualitative patterns of self-awareness) that vary from one person to another.

Transformation in Adulthood Dimensions

If we consider Western knowledge as a whole as if it were the temporal becoming of an individual knowing organization, it shows characteristics of an orthogenetic progression whose directionality is distinctly oriented toward a progressive increase of individuation and self-awareness. From its beginnings, the crucial hallmark of Western experience has been the enacting of the self in the process of explaining it (Johnson, 1985) to the point where the individual has gradually come to identify him- or herself with his or her individual consciousness rather than with belonging to a pre-established cosmic order. The primacy of the "psychological dimension" has gradually been assumed in the course of the last century, and in no other era has there been found a level of structural complexity in individual consciousness such as that which is characteristic of our time (Aries & Duby, 1987; Braudel, 1979). Such radical changes deserve mention in that they play an important role in the nature and dynamics of personal reorganization that characterize our experience of adulthood.

In the first place, the contemporary sense of self differs markedly not only from that of the last century but even from that of the last generation, especially in the sense that it is experienced as less permanent and more flexible than traditional models. The increased complexity in individual consciousness has made possible a multifaceted experiencing of self inside the continuous sense of sameness, widening the possibilities of abstract self-referring and, therefore, of assimilation of experience. What is more, the perception of a many-sided self has intensified the oscillatory tension between maintenance and change processes, requiring a continual shifting of the point of equilibrium. Personal experience has thus taken the form of an ongoing process of an ever-evolving but unified self (Giele, 1980), in which the perturbing mutability perceived in one's continuity is matched by the ability to go beyond "old identities" and to build up new ones. This existential dimension transpires from the everyday understanding of life tacitly reflected by current products of our culture; writing his impressions to a friend about a film he had just finished, François Truffaut, who always took such care in portraying the sentiments and experiences of our age, noted that: "In the course of life, we become many different people, and it is precisely this that makes memoires seem strange. One person, the latest, strains to unify all the preceding characters" (1988, p. 243).

The experience of selfhood as a continued and evolving process of personal growth has made it possible for awareness of self to take on an increasingly important role as regulator, absolutely crucial in the unfolding of individual lifespan.

Awareness of our actions makes our actions objects of our reflections, and opens their consequences to our liking or disliking of them. Awareness of our liking or disliking of the consequences of what we do makes us aware that we always do what we do because we want the consequences of what we are aware that we do, even when we claim that we do not want those consequences. In other words, awareness of our liking or disliking of the consequences of what we do, constitutes our responsibility because it makes us aware that we do what we do because we want the consequences of what we do. Finally, awareness of our liking or disliking of our liking or disliking of the consequences of what we do, constitutes our human freedom by making us responsible for our emotions through being aware of them, as well as for our liking or disliking them in our actions. In the recursive involvement between languaging, emotioning and becoming, that our epigenesis entails, we human beings live our lives in a continuous recursive involvement between awareness and becoming. In these circumstances it is not the same for us to be aware or not to be aware of what we do in our interpersonal relations, and it is not the same for our body dynamics in all its dimensions, because the courses that our lives follow in our continuous body change and transformation, are at every instant contingent to our awareness, or lack of awareness, of our actions. We can be aware of this now. (Maturana, 1988a, p. 81)

However, the experience of life as continued personal growth is likely to set up a positive feedback toward higher degrees of internal complexity which may prove critical. Firstly, managing the perceived changeability of one's continuity requires good levels of cognitive and emotive flexibility and entails a progressive increase in self-consciousness. Secondly, the rise in self-consciousness is paralleled by a growing perception of ambiguity in the current appraisal of self that triggers unbalancing emotions such as boredom, a sense of absurdity, and so on, increasing, in the final analysis, the demand for flexibility.

Moreover, the changed appraisal of the self has set off a consistent transformation in the ideology of love, which has profoundly modified the role of affective relationships in adulthood as well as the way of experiencing them (Smelser, 1980; Swidler, 1980).

Love is still central in the search for self-knowledge, but this search is no longer identified as a single, decisive choice which will bear a life commitment. Quite the contrary, love comes gradually to be conceived of as a continuous process of personal growth and self-identification taking place within a whole sequence of relationships and facing one crisis after another. In addition, while previously the obstacles to reaching a stable life commitment were identified as external factors against which one could only rebel or give up, now the obstacles to love are experienced as internal to the self and to the relationship, so that the struggle for deepening communication and for discovering "real" aspects of the self have become the main ingredients of our love experience.

> In the shifting structure of the love myth, the impulsive sides of the self are given greater emphasis, and the ideal of permanence is undermined. What is good about a relationship is not the commitment it embodies, but how much a person learns about himself from the relationship. Love is not the emblem of a crystallized identity but the mandate for continuing self-exploration. In the traditional view, a love that ended was a failure, a sign of some terrible mistake in the search for self and identity. But the new love imagery can claim great gains from failed relationships. (Swidler, 1980, p. 129)

Thus, in the affective realm too, flexibility (i.e., the ability to take up and leave close relationships) can help the subject manage disrupting emotions, so influencing, to a large extent, his or her capacity for further development. It should also be noted that this change in the experience of love, while on the one hand making the sense of personal identity much more flexible and generative, has, on the other, increased the importance of the processes of separation and grieving, lending to this increased self-flexibility a component of emotional instability that surely plays a role in the existential crisis of contemporary humankind.

II

PSYCHOTHERAPEUTIC PRINCIPLES

It happens in reality, as much in personal life as in history, that only in certain exceptional moments does doing correspond to willing. Indeed, what characterizes human experience is exactly the twofold necessity underlying any action: on the one hand required by circumstance, to meet that challenge which circumstance is continually casting before Man and to which he must respond even at the cost of being annihilated; and on the other hand, required by his own internal condition; it is exactly here that the tragedy of human experience lies: every man knows himself, even before thinking, as doing and carrying out; *he knows after he has acted.* When he does something, that which most answers his passions, his longings, he does it without knowing that he is doing so.
    —M. ZAMBRANO, *Persona y Democracia* (1958/1988, pp. 62–63)

5

A Post-Rationalist Framework for Cognitive Therapy

PRELIMINARY REMARKS

The ontological approach that we have attempted to outline thus far entails a remarkable transformation in the conceptualization of change and therapeutic methodology with respect to the current rationalist perspective (Guidano, 1987, 1988; Mahoney, 1984, 1985, 1988, 1991; Mahoney & Lyddon, 1988; Mahoney, Lyddon, & Arfold, 1989). The most important aspects of this transformation may be outlined as follows (Guidano, 1991).

In traditional cognitive approaches, which still regard knowledge as the representation of an objective and univocal order that exists independently from our being in the world, emotional disturbances derive from an insufficiently valid correspondence between individual beliefs and external reality; that is, unpleasant feelings are merely indicative of distorted thinking in accordance with the well-known saying: "as you think, so shall you feel." Thus, because the assessment is aimed at identifying "wrong" beliefs and irrational automatic thoughts, comparing the client's behavior with a set of standard rational axioms taken as universally valid, the basic principle of change revolves around this theme: in order to modify perturbing emotions, it is sufficient to change the corresponding "irrational" beliefs as these gradually come to light.

A rational supremacy of this kind results in the establishment of a self-control strategy centered on *persuasion:* the therapist tries with every available means to convince the client to endorse more rational

93

beliefs and to enact more convenient attitudes, while instructing him or her to control and/or eliminate the effects of negative emotions. The most suitable operational setting for such a procedure is a more or less pressing dialectical confrontation in which the therapist plays the role of "enlightened sage," "devil's advocate," or "hidden persuader" according to his or her personal background and professional training. Persuasion, in turn, technically consists of intervening at the surface structure level (imagery, internal dialogue, beliefs, etc.), directed at modifying the semantic aspects of explicit cognitive processes, while neglecting the tacit syntactic rules which are at the base of these processes.

In agoraphobic subjects, while basic syntactic rules maintain clients' perceptions of themselves as defenseless in a menacing, hostile world, the intervention is focused, for instance, on the way they represent to themselves a panic attack in the traffic, accompanied by a series of instructions that they must introduce in their inner dialogue whenever they again face the feared situation. No doubt clients will obtain better control over anxiety in feared situations if they keep telling themselves: "I must remember the doctor told me nothing can happen to me . . .," "I must keep calm, it's all my imagination . . .," "Nobody ever died from waiting at a traffic light. . . ." Undeniably, though, the meaning of anxiety attacks remains unchanged for clients, and furthermore, they still have no explanation for their being so "strangely" oversensitive and vulnerable to unimportant situations of constriction and/or loneliness. If the intervention is limited to a modification of the cognitive appraisal, the perturbing emotional reaction is in no way changed in tone, even though its intensity can be better controlled (Zajonc, 1984). Critical emotions remain alien to the subject who, instead, has acquired skills in controlling them "from the outside." Thus, rather than a reorganization of personal meaning, what has occurred is only a semantic change inside the same meaning tonality.

Moreover, given that the aim is to make the client's behavior fit with a set of rational axioms, the therapist is frequently driven to induce more adaptive attitudes through relational or cognitive-behavioral maneuvers (paradoxical prescriptions, challenging dialectic disconfirmations, etc.) which almost completely exclude the client's self-awareness, that is, the comprehension of his or her way of experiencing and explaining self and reality. In other words, if the perspective endorsed is centered on an objective, immutable outside

order that unequivocally rules the trend and sense of human events, the therapeutic relationship cannot become other than an instrument, and a more or less authoritarian one, for the reestablishment of that order—rather than a facilitator for clients' personal explorations in finding a path for their gradual understanding of the rules that constrain the rigid coherence of their personal meaning, through the apparent senselessness of their disturbing emotions.

On the other hand, if the ordering of reality into personal experience is, ontologically, a self-referent construction, we cannot expect to identify any objective outside point of view from which to evaluate the degree of rationality and validity of the problematic behavior exhibited. Rather than being an absolute criterion for judging an attitude in itself, rationality is instead intrinsically relativistic and, as such, simply permits a definition of the degree of adequacy of a given attitude *if the latter is referred to the specific personal meaning that generated it and to which it belongs.*

From an evolutionary point of view, rationality appears to be an emerging property of self-organizing systems and from the beginning it is connected to the development of more and more effective purpose-directed behavior. Hence if rationality is interwoven with the experience of acting, it cannot refer solely to the logical-abstract categories (true–false) employed in reordering such experience semantically (Weimer, 1987). In other words, rationality merely highlights the self-referentiality of adaptive processes in a given system, and adaptation itself consists not so much of attaining a "right" or "true" purpose (validity), as pursuing an aim whose usefulness is only possible from the internal point of view of the system involved (viability).

In terms of the ontological perspective being presented, we can thus say that through the continuous process of reordering immediate experiencing ("I") into a conscious sense of self and the world ("Me"), every subject is able to structure a stable, and at the same time, dynamic demarcation between what is real and what is not in his or her ongoing praxis of living. In this sense, clients' attainment of a more articulated and exhaustive *comprehension* of their functioning represents the crucial variable for assimilating extraneous and unpleasant feelings perceived as "unreal," and transforming them into "real" personal emotions, that is, a reorganization of immediate experiencing ("I") in which negative affect can be self-referred and abstracted into one's conscious sense of continuity and uniqueness ("Me").

As is thus evident, an ontological, process-oriented approach conceptualizes feelings and affect as forms of knowing in and of themselves, that is, as the immediate ordering of reality that we experience *a priori* in our ongoing praxis of living. On the one hand, the continuous emotional modulation provided by recurrent and oscillative psychophysiological patterns integrates past, present, and anticipated experiences; on the other hand, the emergence of discrepant feelings out of such modulation is the essential requisite for triggering reorganizations in the patterns of coherence which regulate the unfolding of personal meaning processes.

On these premises, we may formulate two general principles about the close connection between affectivity and change in the process of psychotherapy:

No change seems possible without emotions.

Throughout lifespan development the continuity and coherence of personal meaning processes rely on the dynamic equilibrium between the organizational unity of the individual's emotional domain ("I") and the conscious self-image ("Me") through which this felt experience is made consistent; the self-regulation between core affective themes provides a focus and direction in organizing the individual's thoughts, feelings, and actions along dimensions of abstract and integrated knowledge compatible with his or her self-awareness. In addition, while ideational themes (i.e., dimensions of abstract knowledge) usually go through a more or less continuous process of differentiation, recombination, and integration, basic affective themes seem much more constant in time and exhibit a different rate and mechanism of change as compared to cognitive structures (cf. Haviland, 1984). The assumption according to which a change in cognition entails a corresponding change in emotions therefore turns out to be groundless, in that self-regulation and self-development of core affective themes seem not to be as influenced by logical rules of differentiation and integration as ideational themes are. In other words, it appears even more evident that *while thinking usually changes thoughts, only feeling can change emotions;* that is, only the emergence of new emotional experiences, resulting from the addition of new tonalities of feelings to the unitary configuration of core emotional themes, can affect self-regulation, modify current patterns of self-perception, and thus facilitate a reordering in personal meaning processes.

The structure and quality of change depend to a large extent on the level and quality of self-awareness with which the subject carries out the reorganization process.

Indeed, far from being a beam of light which reveals an already well arranged and complete configuration of elements, merely acknowledging their presence, self-awareness is a constructive self-referent ordering that determines to a large extent the form that personal experience will assume. As an example, a "personal revolution"—that is, a successful deep change (Mahoney, 1980)—and a clear-cut clinical syndrome—that is, an unsuccessful deep change—although both triggered by a deep emotional perturbation, are the outcomes of different explicit reordering processes, which in turn result from different qualitative levels of self-awareness and abstract thought. Thus, a viable assimilation of perturbing feelings necessarily requires a change in the "Me" appraisal of the experiencing "I," and so it is necessary to trigger progressive shifts in current patterns of self-awareness by increasing clients' comprehension of the way in which they order ongoing experience. Both clinical and basic research should therefore be more preferentially oriented toward (1) the study of variables (developmental patterns of immediate experience, self-referring concreteness/abstractness levels, etc.) that underlie the structuring of self-awareness in an individual lifespan; and (2) the study of the relationship existing between the individual's level and quality of self-awareness and the possible ways in which he or she can reorder meaning coherence.

How are the above considerations reflected by the general methodology of a nonrationalistic, process-oriented cognitive therapy?

In the first place, the crucial operational setting lies at the interface between immediate experiencing and its explicit reordering; the basic procedure consists of training clients, through self-observation techniques, to differentiate between immediate self-perception and conscious beliefs and attitudes, and then to reconstruct the patterns of coherence that they follow in making what they feel consistent.

Secondly, for such a strategy to be effective, the client must gradually experience during the therapeutic process some affect-laden events which can progressively exert pressure in the direction of reorganization (Greenberg & Safran, 1987; Safran & Greenberg, 1991). Throughout the process, the therapist must be able to provide tools of analysis and self-observation which, by increasing the flexibility and plasticity of clients' levels of self-awareness, will enable them to gradually accomplish a progressive reordering of personal experience—one where the problematic perturbation is assimilated and understood in a more abstract and integrated self-image, not involving any particular emotional distress.

Finally, the therapeutic relationship is the specific context in which it becomes possible for the therapist both to set off affective change events and to guide the reorganization process that they activate. The therapeutic relationship is for all intents and purposes a *real, living interaction,* and its emotional aspects produce a facilitating effect for the assimilation of new experiences or the reframing of existing ones.

To give more specifically articulated form to these observations, let us go on to outline the most important aspects inherent in the therapeutic methodology and strategy.

THE THERAPIST'S ATTITUDE AND THE ASSESSMENT PROCEDURE

As one would expect in a perspective of this kind, the therapist's attitude in the clinical setting is considerably different from traditional approaches.

Within a therapeutic relationship intended to be essentially a tool of exploration, the therapist will scrupulously avoid confronting the perturbing emotions with a critical and/or worried attitude which would inevitably confirm for the client the sense of extraneousness with which he or she usually perceives such emotions, and would thus further decrease the possibility of their assimilation. Moreover, since the aim consists not so much of modifying the client's beliefs at any cost, but rather of facilitating him or her to become aware of his or her way of elaborating beliefs, the therapist orients, from the very beginning, the client's comprehension toward his or her basic patterns for self-referring immediate experience. Thus, by gradually reconstructing the internal coherence existing beneath the apparent extraneousness of disturbing feelings, the therapist makes the client realize with growing clarity how such emotions contain fundamental information, the understanding of which will very likely facilitate further comprehension of the current existential stalemate.

On the other hand, in order for the therapist to be in a position to maintain such an attitude, it is indispensable that, as part of his or her professional experience, he or she should know the dynamics of the principal organizations of personal meanings (P. M. Orgs.; see Chapter 3) as well as the lifespan developmental challenges that are encountered in their orthogenetic progression.

Negative affects (anxiety, sadness, helplessness, etc.) are part of the range of feeling tonalities with which humans experience their environment. However, the same tonality (e.g., anxiety) may be ordered and experienced in very different ways (e.g., connected to loss, danger, lack of certainty) according to whether it forms part of a pattern of depressive, phobic, or obsessive meaning coherence. The same may be said for more interpersonally structured affect, such as the fear of negative judgments from others, which all humans, as intersubjective animals, exhibit in their emotional repertoire. However, for an eating disorders organization, the perception of negative judgment is matched by an even more blurred and wavering sense of self; in a depressive organization, it triggers a loss reaction and grieving; in a phobic organization, it is felt as a threat to the need for protection, and so on.

Indeed, adherence to a process-oriented model of personal meaning development makes the therapist less externally bound to current problems, and allows him or her to use them to foster new levels of comprehension, thus allowing the self-organization processes of the client to influence the direction of the therapy. Rationalists appear more externally bound to the immediate and concrete aspects exhibited by current symptoms and tend to guide the course of the therapy according to moment-to-moment presentation of problems and specific goals (Mahoney & Lyddon, 1988).

This does not mean "pigeon-holing" the client from the start, applying a static "diagnostic label," as inevitably happens when the descriptive nosography expressed by the DSM-III-R is adopted, or when use is made of lists of critical beliefs supposed to be specific of anxiety, depression, etc.

In the first place, the notion of a P.M.Org. is not to be regarded as an entity made up of specific knowledge *contents* which can be defined once and for all; rather, it is a unitary and self-organized ordering of meaning invariants capable of structuring a wide variety of possible knowledge contents, the coherence of which can be grasped only by focusing on the *processing* modalities (flexibility, abstraction, integration) with which its meaning dimension unfolds throughout the lifespan. Finally, although inevitably coming under the categories of meaning within which the human experience of life is included, each person is a *unique* experiment of Nature and thus has an absolutely unique way of articulating both his or her meaning dimension and the reordering processes that take place within it.

It is undoubtedly advisable to preface discussion of assessment by pointing out that it is a little specious to talk of it as if it were something unto itself. It is in fact part of a complex and multidirectional process, psychotherapy, which unfolds simultaneously at several levels all closely interwoven but irreducible one to another. In particular, it is almost impossible to differentiate assessment from intervention. Actually, the assessment is carried out at the experiencing/explaining interface through the self-observational skills that the client is gradually developing and, therefore, as we shall later see, is inherently linked to the ongoing reordering process. Our aim will therefore be simply to outline the essential methodological aspects.

The crucial feature characterizing the therapist's attitude in the assessment procedure is constituted by the ability to differentiate between immediate experiencing (i.e., what is happening in one's praxis of living) and its explanation (i.e., making it consistent with one's self-conception). It is certainly not an easy attitude to adopt as the therapist is dealing with the well-known problem of distinguishing fact from theory; this is a fundamental methodological problem regarding scientific knowledge in its entirety, and which, although an essential problem, continues to be controversial, as is well exemplified by Ritter (1979):

> . . . I often have the impression that scientists forget what is fact and what is theory. The frequency of light waves, for example, has been associated with the experience of color. Some scientists seem to think that light waves constitute the real world and the conscious experiences of color associated with them some kind of unreliable, shadow events. But it is the light waves which are hypothetical (no one has ever seen them). Color is a fact. Scientific theories are held with varying degrees of confidence, and an essential tenet of science is that theories can in principle never be entirely proven. Such is not the case with conscious experience. That we experience color is not an idea to be held with varying degrees of confidence: it is a fact of human

existence. Indeed, all conscious experiences are facts and represent the only things we can be certain of. (p. 208)

In other words, the point to bear in mind is that the "facts" correspond to the client's immediate experiencing (as in the case of color experience) while his or her explaining/reasoning are ways for self-referring facts in order to make them understandable (as in the case of light waves). As a consequence, while assessing a given situation (e.g., a marital quarrel), the therapist should not focus on the way in which the client talks about what happened; quite the contrary, while reconstructing the event with the same meticulousness with which one would reconstruct a scene from a film, he or she should be able to continually shift his or her focus from one level to the other:

1. How the client's experience happened in the situation (e.g., perception of discrepancy in the spouse's attitude, in what way the discrepany was felt in order to trigger anger, the experience of anger and related feelings, the emotional effects of becoming aware of being angry).
2. How the client self-refers and explains what is happening in the situation (e.g., contingent reasons adopted for the quarrel which exclude, or at least reduce, responsibility for it; explanations of his or her aggressive style in terms of personality traits or dispositions; inferences about intentions and moods of the spouse).

A basic distinction between the two levels is that the latter has truth value while the former does not. In other words, immediate experiencing simply expresses the inescapable way of being-in-the-world and, as such, can never be mistaken, whereas explanations, belonging to a semantic meta-level, can be erroneous when compared to the experience they are intended to explain. Thus, in the quarrel example, even if the explanations and reasons adopted turn out to be irrelevant and inconsistent with respect to the experiential situation, the therapist should not limit him- or herself to criticism of the irrationality of certain attitudes, and suggestions for more suitable ones. Actually, experiencing anger as a response to minimal triggers is an important indication, and should lead the therapist to a more profound investigation of the structure of the relationship and the quality of the emotional reciprocity.

Proceeding in the assessment by alternately focusing on the client's immediate experiencing and his or her explanations, the therapist continually deals with direct (verbal/nonverbal behavior) and indirect (reports of events) observational data. The therapist should bear in mind that such data, as well as being closely interwoven, appear to be so interdependent that they reciprocally influence and specify each other. This interdependence can be schematized as follows:

Effect of direct data on indirect ("What happened is said now"). The way in which a past event is related (e.g., gestures, semantic patterns used, emotional modulation) and the moment in the therapeutic relationship at which the client decides to relate it (e.g., oscillations in approach–avoidance balance, need for a greater involvement in the relationship) provide a preunderstanding which helps the therapist grasp the meaning tacitly attributed by the client to the event, and this, in the final analysis, further clarifies the report itself.

Effect of indirect data on direct ("What is said now is influenced by what happened in the past"). The way in which the client manages the reorganization he or she is going through (type of resistance to change) as well as the client's emotional position within the therapeutic setting (e.g., fears expressed, reassurances requested, affective guarantees expected) allow a glimpse of the client's attachment history and developmental trajectory, and this in turn helps the therapist grasp the meaning tacitly endorsed by the client in the ongoing therapeutic interpersonal context.

Focusing alternately on experiencing and explaining and using moment-to-moment the interdependence between direct and indirect data should thus be considered basic methodological aspects of the assessment procedure, both in the initial phases, when reconstructing the patterns of coherence underlying the problematic behavior exhibited, and in more advanced phases, when assessment of the client's past history aids in the reconstruction of the developmental pathway that has led to such patterns.

There is one final difference with respect to the attitudes of proponents of other approaches toward resistance. In the rationalist view, resistances are considered indicators of motivational deficits (e.g., irrational fears, ambivalence, approach–avoidance conflict) which must be overcome, whereas in an ontological and constructivistic approach, resistances correspond to self-referent mechanisms for maintaining current patterns of internal coherence in spite of the pressures to reorder them. Hence resistances and self-regulation are intertwined with self-deceiving patterns to slow down and/or distort the assimilation of critical data, reflecting natural processes which protect the individual from changing too much, too quickly; they should be worked "with" rather than "against" (Bugental & Bugental, 1984; Mahoney, 1991). Finally, as Mahoney and Lyddon (1988) remark, respect for the implicit wisdom of these systemic processes is more likely to facilitate progressive psychological development than attempts to deny their significance or to constrain their expression.

SELF-OBSERVATION METHOD

Self-observation is the essential method for carrying on both the assessment and the intervention, insofar as it permits the reconstruction of events of therapeutic interest, working at the interface between immediate experiencing and its explicit reordering. It permits, in this way, the analysis of both levels of processing as well as the relationship existing between them. In this sense, therefore, self-observation is clearly differentiated both from introspection (e.g., free-association technique) where the first level is privileged, and from self-monitoring techniques (e.g., detection of automatic thoughts) where the explicit level is privileged. The essential aspects of the method and the basic instructions given to the client are as follows:

First of all, one must always start with an event or a series of events which may then be analyzed one by one. Any problem presented by a client may be reformulated in terms of the events that produced it and to which it refers.

Adopting a kind of "cinematographic language," which, because of its immediate comprehensibility, simplifies the instructions and makes them less boring, the therapist reconstructs with the client the succession of scenes making up the event under investigation. Then, as if one were in an editing room, the client is trained to "pan" the succession of scenes, going back and forth in slow motion, to "zoom in" on a single scene to focus on particular aspects, to "zoom out," reinserting the same scene enriched with new details back into the sequence, and so on ("moviola technique"). Clearly, whenever a scene enriched with details is reinserted in the sequence, the latter mutates, taking on new connotations, permitting the emergence of further details in other scenes.

scene 1 . . . scene 2 . . . scene 3 . . . scene n
<u>Zooming in/out</u>

Panning

As can be seen, the basic procedure is relatively simple; it is clear, however, that self-observation is essentially a method and can be carried out at even more structured levels as one proceeds through the phases of the therapy and the client's self-observational skills become more efficient and articulated.

In the initial phases of the therapy, where it is necessary to guide the client to an understanding and appreciation of the differentiation between immediate experiencing and his or her self-referring and explaining it, the basic scene analysis consists of reconstucting (1) the patterns of immediate experiencing that occurred in the situation putting into focus the entire way of happening of the client in the scene (e.g., mimicry, gesture, posture, "reverse" or "unwilled" actions, meaningful omissions, emotional role assumed in the interpersonal context); and (2) the emotions consciously self-referred as the client experiences the situation, and the interpretation rules by which that situation called forth those emotions. These aspects can be reconstructed directly from the client's reports.

Naturally, in addition to considering how they talk to themselves or others about their emotions and how they conceptualize them after the event, clients should be suitably trained to focus on the structure of their immediate experience that occurred in the course of the situation. A simple way to do this is to point out that in investigating an emotional experience there are two types of questions one can ask: (1) the *why* of that experience, which yields data on how a person self-refers and self-explains what has been felt, and (2) the *how* of the composition of what was felt, that is, its structure (e.g., imagery modulation, basic affect tonalities and related feelings, sense of self). Assuming that the therapist is able to make this differentiation in his or her own emotional experiences, he or she, proceeding through the scene-analysis procedure, should guide clients in shifting their point of view from the "why" to the "how," while reconstructing the type of difficulty experienced by them in such shifting.

The moment this differentiation gets under way, the client can begin to see him- or herself from two alternate points of view: while carrying out a given scene in the first person ("subjective viewpoint"), and while looking at oneself in that scene from without ("objective viewpoint"). The client's flexibility in subjective/objective differentiation further improves the possibilities of reconstruction of the immediate experience, given that, from an objective viewpoint, the client is now able to make inferences about the possible structure of the subjective viewpoint experienced in the situation. This is more or less what takes place when one thinks and talks about a scene from a film: starting with the words and actions of a character, one tries to reconstruct the moods, affective motivations, secret intentions, and so on. The difference is that the person one is trying to reconstruct is oneself.

This same procedure can also be used in the more advanced phases of the therapy when reconstruction of developmental history is being undertaken (infancy and preschool years, childhood, adolescence, and youth); because of the client's advanced skills, the reconstruction of the subjective viewpoint with which the event was experienced at a certain age can be carried out from two different objective viewpoints: (1) as one would have seen oneself from without at that same age, and (2) as one sees oneself now from without while focusing on that age.

As can be seen, rather than the modification of ways of thinking judged to be erroneous, the essential aspect of the self-observation method consists of clients' gradual acquisition of an appreciable degree of flexibility in assessing their selfhood dynamics because of the ability, on the one hand, to differentiate their experiencing "I" from the appraising "Me," and, on the other, to be able to see the whole process from both a subjective and an objective viewpoint.

Both the increase in emotional openness and self-revelation (better focusing on immediate experience) and the possibility of being able to see oneself objectively from without inevitably modify the current sense of self (Clark & Reis, 1988; Csikszentmihalyi & Figurski, 1982; Miall, 1986). Moreover, repeatedly viewing the same affect-laden scene in slow motion, going back and forth from many points of view, brings about a modification of the way it is appraised and self-referred, with a consequent change in the current relationship between "episodic" and "semantic" memory (see Tulving, 1972, 1985); all this inevitably becomes translated into a reframing of the same scene which triggers the emergence of other feeling tonalities.

Hence, while such flexibility increases, the usual viewpoint on oneself ("Me") is gradually challenged, so that new aspects of the experiencing "I" can come into the picture.

Therefore, the basic therapeutic effect resulting from an increasing flexibility in selfhood dynamics consists of a gradual changing in the "Me" appraisal of the "I" matched by a consistent degree of emotional restructuring; that is, new feeling tonalities in one's ongoing immediate experiencing are recognized and self-referred, thus becoming essential ingredients in one's perceived range of conscious emotions.

Finally, the self-observation method can gradually be directed toward another basic modification in selfhood dynamics: an increased flexibility about others' perspective taking. The attainment of such flexibility is particularly important in those clinical situations in which there is a marked vulnerability to others' judgments, both actual and anticipated.

As we have seen (see Part I), we live in an intersubjective dimension, so that from the very beginning each of us develops a conscious sense of self ("Me") for making ongoing immediate experience ("I") consistent which is closely correlated to how one perceives others seeing one.

In a healthy developmental pathway, the self–nonself differentiation achieves a stable and defined demarcation from others, so that the subject sets his or her ongoing continuity and sameness as the point of reference in self-organizing his or her experience with others while interacting with them. Any pattern of immediate experiencing ("I") which is recognized and self-referred as a dimension of the conscious self ("Me") becomes, simultaneously, a tool for recognizing the same dimension in others, while the perceived difference stimulates the search for new patterns in one's ongoing immediate experience. In other words, the subject is "internally bound" in self-defining, so that information coming from interactions with others is mainly used to understand people as separate persons, autonomous in their thinking and feeling.

In contrast, in a developmental pathway in which the self–nonself differentiation has been poor (see Chapter 3, eating disorders organization), a sense of self is mainly constructed with the expectations perceived in others, and consequently the "Me" results from assuming the perspectives of significant others. The experiencing "I" therefore becomes recognizable and self-referable to the extent to which its patterns of emotional modulation fit with the perspectives perceived in others. That is, the subject is "externally bound" and derives the definition of him- or herself from the behavior and attitudes of others, as if they were a mirror. This state of things, apart from showing patterns of emotional overreactivity linked to the perception of noncorrespondence with others' expectations (oversensitivity to others' judgments), also makes it possible that others are never seen as autonomous persons, but only as confirmation or disconfirmation of the current sense of self, and are thus always magnified positively or negatively.

The self-observational procedure has shown itself to be most useful in triggering a modification of the viewpoint on oneself (i.e., a change in the "Me" appraisal of the "I") linked to a concomitant modification of how others are seen. After the initial phase, necessary in order that clients may grasp the experiencing/explaining differentiation and see themselves alternately from a subjective and objective viewpoint, they are trained, in the "moviola technique," to see the same affect-laden scene with a significant other alternately from two different viewpoints:

1. Perceiving others' behavior as information about oneself (e.g., "If A behaves that way, what about me? Who am I?").
2. Perceiving others' behavior as information about them (e.g., "If A behaves that way, what about him or her? Who is he or she?").

The first goal consists of making the client realize that these different types of attribution correspond to totally different dimensions of oneself and reality. In subsequent steps, through the scene analysis of relevant interactional events, the therapist guides the client in shifting his or her viewpoint on others, while at the same time assessing and reconstructing the difficulties inherent in such shifting.

We are here dealing with a self-observational procedure that should be used in all circumstances linked to problems connected with eating disorders P.M.Orgs., where the attunement to the perceived judgment of others may reach the point of a true sense of self-annihilation. However, as sensitivity to the judgment of others is typical of human experience, one may often also come up against this hypersensitivity in other P.M.Orgs., which, even if it is less intense and has a different meaning, may still become a source of perturbing feelings in ongoing interpersonal relationships. Given that the sensitivity to judgment is based on taking the behavior of others as information about oneself, this same method can also be used in these circumstances.

STRUCTURE AND DYNAMICS
OF THERAPEUTIC CHANGE

In a therapeutic perspective centered on the reorganization of personal meaning, a significant therapeutic modification coincides with a change in the "Me" appraisal of the experiencing "I"—that is, a change of the current viewpoint on oneself—and this involves a deeper recognition and appreciation of aspects of immediate ex- periencing which, although extremely affect laden, had been ne- glected up to that moment (Greenberg, 1984; Safran & Greenberg, 1991; Guidano, 1987, 1988; Mahoney, 1991).

Basically, a change in the "Me" appraisal of the "I" consists of a shifting from experiencing some aspect in one's praxis of living as "objectively given"—and not deserving further reflection—to self- referring and appraising it as a dynamic way of explaining and validat- ing one's being-in-the-world, and as such, subject to further inquiry and reflection upon its origin. In other words, whenever the "given" is broken, it can be relativized and traced back to the system of selfhood demarcations and distinctions (Habermas, 1979). Naturally, there is a range of possible shiftings distributed across different levels of com- plexity and structural order. However, the occurrence of any shifting necessarily requires the parallel emergence of a more inclusive order- ing process, which should be made available through the therapeutic setting. For each possible shifting there is a corresponding level of ordering process, the attainment of which makes the shifting possible. Far from being a merely cognitive phenomenon, the emergence of more inclusive ordering levels ("meta-cognition" or "knowing about knowing") is a complex process of integration between sensorimotor- ic, affective, and conceptual ingredients; therefore, its emergence into consciousness is always matched by a sense of ambiguity resulting from the discrepancy experienced in one's previous level of ordering pro- cesses (Hayek, 1978; Guidano, 1987; Mahoney, 1985, 1991).

Different degrees of change are possible, capable of triggering reorganizations of personal experience of varying depth and articulation; as a result, the notion of "superficial" and "deep" changes introduced by Arnkoff (1980) and Mahoney (1980) has become accepted in cognitive therapy. The two types of change are not mutually exclusive; quite the contrary, as we shall see, they may be part of different stages in the same psychotherapeutic process, and often a superficial change in the initial phases of the therapy may facilitate the attainment of a deeper change in more advanced stages.

It is important to emphasize that there is *no* direct correlation between the type of strategic intervention carried out and the quality of change processes which occur, even though it is clear that therapeutic intervention has in some way triggered the process that brought about reorganization. In other words, the therapist can only try to set forth "conditions" capable of triggering a reorganization, but cannot determine nor control either when clients reorganize or the final outcome of the reorganization (Dell & Goolishian, 1981; Guidano, 1987). These "conditions" essentially consist of the production of affect-laden events capable of modifying immediate experiencing in such a way that the client cannot avoid recognizing and self-referring it (change of the "Me" appraisal of the "I"). The emotional perturbations capable of triggering affective change events in the course of the therapeutic process derive from two basic sources:

1. The increase in clients' comprehension of their rules of functioning is always paralleled by an appreciable degree of emotional modulation in which new tonalities of feelings are likely to emerge. On the other hand, modifications in clients' comprehension in some way derive from the explanations offered by the therapist, and obviously, anything the therapist says or does can be considered an explanation, the training in the self-observation method included.
2. The structure and reciprocity of the therapeutic interpersonal context can also trigger emotional perturbations which facilitate the challenging of clients' current viewpoints on themselves.

The attempt to exhaustively conceptualize the close correlation between affective events and change processes has led me to pose the problem in these terms (Guidano, 1991). The essential requisite facilitating a therapeutic change appears to be the simultaneous unfolding of two processes, the intensity and structure of which range widely: (1) a *discrepant effect* (deriving from the explanations set forth by the therapist) which is able to trigger off an appreciable modification of the viewpoint the client entertains about him- or herself, and (2) a consistent level of *emotional involvement* in the therapeutic relationship. A deeper analysis of these processes may help to clarify their reciprocal correlation.

The efficacy of therapeutic explanations and interpretations depends on the degree of discrepancy perceived by clients between them and their usual sense of themselves (Claiborn, 1982; Claiborn & Dowd, 1985). Thus, in contrast to the traditional assumption, the crucial effect, rather than being identified with the transmission of more rational knowledge content, can be traced back to the emergence of perturbing feelings that provoke a reappraisal of the client's immediate experiencing. Such reappraisal, in turn, involves a modification of the current level of self-awareness, the constructive and generative effect of which unfolds through a reordering of the configuration of items contained in the client's self-image. However, even though the availability of explanations conveying discrepant effects is a necessary condition for activating a challenging perturbation, it is not sufficient in itself for triggering a reorganizing effect.

An appreciable level of emotional involvement in the therapeutic relationship renders the client unable to avoid facing a challenging point of view, constraining him or her to an immediate and global self-referent encoding that generates the perception of discrepancy. In other words, regardless of its specific content, a challenging perspective can produce a discrepant effect only through the level of self-referentiality that it acquires as a function of the quality of emotional reciprocity thus far structured in the interpersonal context. As common experience shows, a message penetrates according to the quality of ongoing interaction. Criticism from someone to whom we are indifferent generally leaves us unperturbed—and often even has a "paradoxically" confirming effect—whereas the same remark from a very significant person is likely to upset us deeply.

However, the necessity for emotional involvement should not concern just the client; the therapist's involvement in the setting exerts a crucial role in activating in the client that condition of unavoidability and self-referentiality previously described. Actually, the centrality of commitment in the structure of language acts— emphasized concomitantly by evolutionary epistemology and onto-

The therapeutic approach which we shall present in the following chapters usually involves weekly sessions. The entire strategy consists of three main phases following in sequence:

- Phase 1: Preparing the clinical and interpersonal context.
- Phase 2: Construing the therapeutic setting.
- Phase 3: Undertaking the developmental analysis.

Psychotherapy is inherently a complex and multidirectional process that unfolds simultaneously across many levels, so the attempt to identify a sequence of phases where in fact there is a network of interwoven processes is an explicatory artifice aimed at exemplifying an operative praxis.

Moreover, given that an essential element of the therapeutic strategy we are about to present is founded on a developmental, process-oriented methodology which conceptualizes psychopathology as a science of personal meaning (see Chapter 3), it is important to give at least an idea of the way in which the main P.M.Orgs. undergo, during the therapeutic process, a reorganization of their meaning coherence. Therefore, in order to provide a unitary and systematic treatment, we shall try to exemplify the above phases, longitudinally reconstructing the therapeutic course of four clinical cases, each corresponding to a specific P.M.Org.

logical approaches to cognition (Reynolds, 1981; Olafson, Maturana, 1978, 1988a)—has become one of the most innov aspects set forth in the last decade by psycholinguistics (Habeı 1981; Winograd, 1980; Winograd & Flores, 1986):

> The essential presupposition for the success of an illocutionar consists in the speaker's entering into a specific *engagement,* so tha hearer can rely on him. An utterance can count as a promise, ¡ tion, request, question or avowal, if and only if the speaker mak offer that he is ready to make good insofar as it is accepted b᷈ hearer. The speaker must engage himself, that is, indicate th᷈ certain situations he will draw certain consequences for ac (Habermas, 1979, p. 61)

The emotional involvement of the therapist in what he or she sa᷈ does, making it evident that he or she considers him- or he᷈ engaged in a *real* relationship, represents the guarantee that therapist is "ready to make good an offer if only it is accepted by hearer"; this, in turn, makes, in the client's eyes, the possibilit reliable one of an alternative explanation and experiencing of hi᷈ her current problems.

The therapeutic perspective that emerges from this way of p ing the problem of change thus delineates the role of the therapist ɛ *strategically oriented perturber,* that is, a professional helper who, pursuing the "technical" task of modifying the client's self-awaren patterns, is extremely alert in using ongoing emotional oscillatic detected in the interpersonal therapeutic context in order to facilitɛ the comprehension in the client of what is being reconstructe However, the structuring of the therapist's role as strategic perturb according to the methodological rules defining scientific knowled᷈ will require that psychotherapeutic research be more and more focus᷈ upon the elaboration of patterns exemplifying how the emotion oscillations that take place during the comprehension of critical iı formation can enhance the assimilation of new data and/or the refram ing of existing ones. Unfortunately, since we are still far from havin attained an exhaustive, ontological theory of mental functioning tha is able to explain the close interdependence between emotioning anɛ cognizing, the therapist's ability in using relational dynamics in orde to facilitate the client's change cannot but remain, for the present a least, more an "art" than a "science."

6 _____

Preparing the Clinical and Interpersonal Context

INTRODUCTORY REMARKS

This is the stage corresponding to the initial sessions, usually the first two or three; especially in collaborative situations this preparation may be completed quickly, even during the first session, while in more demanding situations, linked to a more or less passive or ambiguous attitude on the part of the client, it may take as many as six to eight sessions.

The outset is generally marked by the classic question: "What problem has brought you here?" While the client is answering, as is usually the case, by laying out his or her clinical picture, the therapist should be in a position to formulate, as early as possible, a hypothesis as to the possible P.M.Org. lying at the base of the symptomatology. Knowing which meaning dimension the client is attempting to act in allows the therapist to obtain an orientation as to the most effective means of reformulating the problem being presented and to avoid the assumption of attitudes which could be inopportune for the client, insofar as they may oppose or be antithetical to his or her coherence. In the cases which we have chosen to exemplify the progress of therapeutic strategy, the situations were presented as follows.

CASE ILLUSTRATIONS

Richard, a 45-year-old writer and film director, gesticulates in a deadpan way and moves very slowly giving a clearly depressed impression. He speaks with apparent difficulty as he relates that for 2 or 3 years he has realized that he has been in a state of dejection and depression from which he feels he is not able to emerge. He is extremely worried because he is neglecting his work and his family (he has a wife and a 13-year-old son) from whom he feels he no longer deserves any affection. What disheartens him most is discovering himself to be "another person" in these last 2 or 3 years, a "weakling," "beaten," who gets frightened by anything, above all by his reactions. In fact, he alternates reactions of intense desperation (from which he cannot hold back) when faced with the most minimal failures or disappointments (e.g., the loss of a tennis match, a friend who puts off an appointment at the last moment) with explosions of uncontrollable rage. He states he is not really aware at the moment of initial anger, which is triggered by negligible opposition, for example, feeling himself to be contradicted while discussing a football match with a friend, or while choosing a television program with his son. Finally, he maintains that he is becoming an impossible person, and will therefore end up, through nobody's fault but his own, alone and abandoned even by those he holds dearest. He notes in passing that at times suicide seems to him to be the only practicable way out, and he ends his exposition in a voice almost choked by the tears he is holding back.

Sandra, a 34-year-old company secretary, married, with a 6-year-old son, arrives at the studio accompanied by her husband who remains in the waiting room during the session.

About 1 year previously, she reports, returning home in her car from work, she had an intense panic attack accompanied by tachycardia and a sense of suffocation, which forced her to stop by the side of the road in total disorientation. Having stopped, she first had the sense of being on the point of fainting, but immediately afterwards was overwhelmed by the fear of losing control, going into a state and being carried off to a psychiatric emergency ward. After she had been parked for about a quarter of an hour, the panic seemed more controllable, and she was able to get home. From that moment, however, she has been afraid both of going out and of staying at home alone or with just her son, so much so that her husband takes her to and collects her from work, and has voluntarily changed his working hours so as to leave her alone at home as little as possible. All this, however, does not reassure her, given that, even with her family around her, she has a constant fear of losing control and committing rash acts (e.g., when she has to use a knife in the kitchen) or giving in to uncontrollable impulses, such as throwing herself from an open window, even though she has no wish to end her life. This last aspect is what frightens her most, and, crying, she repeats that ". . . it's as if I don't recognize myself anymore, not having any control over myself"; she then asks for repeated reassurances as to the "curability" of her "illness" while referring to all kinds of pharmacological treatments she has tried without success. Prompted by the therapist, who asks for clarification of the period immediately preceding the onset of the disturbance, she says that 5 months previously she had had an abortion (wanted by her husband) and that in the following month her mother had suddenly died of a heart attack in her presence. She starts crying again, saying she still feels and will always feel the absence of her mother ". . . because it was the only pure, disinterested affection I had . . . now I have lost that, it's as if nothing else in the world can protect me. . . ."

Winnie, an 18-year-old girl attending the final year of high school, lives at home with her parents, both clerical workers, and a sister 3 years younger.

About 10 months previously, at the end of the summer holiday and of a week-long flirtation, she had gone on a diet because, even though slightly underweight for her size, she felt "ugly" and "fat." In the space of about a week this had turned into an acute anorexic reaction, with amenorrhea, motor hyperactivity, etc. There followed visits to the family doctor who dispensed vitamins and the usual advice. About a month later the situation returned to normal, primarily because of insistent pressure from her mother. Although continuing to be amenorrheic, Winnie began eating almost regular amounts, preferring, however, to eat alone so as to avoid being at the table with her parents, in fact staying alone in her room for hours at a time. From the start of the academic year, there was a sudden drop in her performance at school; this was unbearable to her, having always been top of the class. She continually considered dropping out of school, but gave in to the pressure of her parents who are in favor of her continuing at all costs. The following April (1 month before making an appointment at our Center) she suddenly experienced a high fever (39°C), internal tremors, gastric contractions, and nausea, and refused food. She was forced to stay away from school for a week, during which all the symptoms disappeared except that of nausea over food. When she started lessons again she spent even more time in her room and limited contact with her family to a minimum.

During the session, Winnie appears lost, as if "emptied," and speaks almost mechanically but impeccably in terms of formal construction. What leaves her most dismayed is just that sense of "being empty" or of "not having any consistency" which is constantly accompanied by the fear of "not being able to feel anything anymore." Indeed, she attributes her progressive isolation from her contemporaries, which in recent months has become almost total, to the fear of discovering that she has neither emotions nor interests.

Gregory is a 25-year-old accountant who lives with his wife, to whom he has been married for a year. For the same period of time he has been working in the office of his father-in-law, also an accountant.

For about 7 or 8 months he has been tormented by the presence of "nasty ideas" on which he is forced to ruminate, at high anxiety levels, for long periods, and which he later feels the need to discuss with someone he can trust, namely, his wife. The "nasty ideas" invariably concern his wife and/or his father-in-law and take the form of "presentiments" of deadly and disfiguring diseases which one of them may catch, or of "revelations" which destroy their moral integrity (e.g., incest between father-in-law and wife, a tendency to prostitution on his wife's part). Although present now and again during the day, these presentiments and revelations intensify to the point of being unbearable in the evening, when, after dinner, he relaxes in front of the television with his wife. Telling these thoughts to his wife is the only way of attenuating the growing horror that he may cause these calamities just by thinking them. Nonetheless, the moment this terror is diminished by his wife's reassurances, he is assailed by "remorse," which also gradually becomes unbearable, for having poisoned his wife's life and for having irreparably damaged a "solid" marriage. The only way of diminishing this anxiety becomes, at that point, the taking of massive doses of tranquilizers or alcohol which soon put him to sleep and ward off all problems. In situations where he feels calmer, such as when he is at home with his parents, he wonders whether he might have let slip some gossip about his wife when they were engaged, and that this, amplifed by inevitable distortions if it is passed on by his parents to the neighbors, might cause even further suffering to his wife. Finally, the fact that the previous month his father-in-law had had a malignant tumor diagnosed on the skin of the nose had thrown him into total panic, convincing him that he was really able to cause irreparable calamities to people dear to him, and this had finally prompted him to consult a therapist.

Although obviously frightened, Gregory remains extremely controlled and composed throughout his exposition; he uses with great competence the technical terms that his various presentiments of illness necessitate and is always careful to point out to the therapist that his "nasty ideas" are quite independent of his will and that they carry no resentment or intolerance toward his wife or father-in-law, who remain the most precious relationships of his life.

There will have been no difficulty in recognizing in the above situations a depressive P.M.Org. (Richard), a phobic P.M.Org. (Sandra), an eating disorder P.M.Org. (Winnie), and finally an obsessive–compulsive P.M.Org. (Gregory). Naturally, this ease of discovery is not always the case, especially when the clinical picture is not so clear and the therapist must rely on the invariant modalities of meaning with which the client constructs his or her mode of self-presentation during the session. For example, a phobic situation may present itself atypically (e.g., a general concern about diseases) or may be masked (e.g., a fear of urinary incontinence as a way of "objectifying" a limitation of movement of which the client is not completely aware). Nonetheless, the therapist can still formulate a hypothesis as to the client's meaning organization by reconstructing from the semantic aspects (contingent beliefs and expectations) the key syntactic rules that give coherence to his or her arguments (need for protection and freedom, dangerous world, etc.).

At this point, faced with the set of disturbances which the client has described, the therapist must reach a *reformulation of the problem presented* in terms that will allow operation at the experiencing/explaining interface (self-observation method), while at the same time excluding any aspect connected to notions of disease (external causal attribution). The basic operation therefore consists of redefining the presented problem as "internal" (i.e., feelings inherent in one's way of being that acquire perturbing qualities because they are not sufficiently recognized or explained) with respect to the "external" definition which, usually, the client experiences and exhibits (i.e., extraneous "symptoms" not connected to his or her way of being).

The therapist should not be concerned with the correctness or truthfulness of the client's affirmations, thus avoiding getting into arguments which will not modify what the client experiences, but which may implicitly define, from the start, the interpersonal context as competitive and purely "verbal."

On the contrary, when working toward a reformulation, the therapist begins by defining the interpersonal context as a reciprocal collaboration and the therapeutic relationship as a tool of exploration for *construing* a comprehension which is *not* at the moment available. In this way, rather than entering into the relative merit of the validity of the *contents* put forward by the client, the therapist instead begins to investigate, together with the client, their overall *meaning*, so trying to construct a point of view, both alternative and involving, which shifts the client's focus onto other aspects of him- or herself.

In other words, the therapist behaves as a strategic perturber right from these very first phases. In fact, both reformulating the problem in terms of "one's own feelings" rather than of "strange disturbances," and defining the therapeutic setting as a committed locale for exploration and comprehension rather than merely as a place for being reassured and provided with technical solutions, are different from the client's usual expectations. Therefore, if the emotional interactive context turns out to be adequate, the perturbing effects of discrepant explanations are likely to modify the viewpoint from which the client presents him- or herself.

In the cases that have just been presented, the process of reformulating clinical and interpersonal contexts proceeded, in rough outline, as follows:

While Richard was presenting his situation, the therapist listened with great attention and participation, asking now and again for clarifications of the painful emotions experienced, but without revealing any worry or perplexity about the despairing conclusions at which the client regularly arrived.

At the end of the exposition, the therapist noted that this "feeling myself to be another person" seemed, at that moment, the aspect to be gone into further, given how much it shocked and depressed him. The therapist therefore began by asking if at other times in the course of his 45 years he had ever felt sensations and moods analogous to this. Richard, as if disconcerted or disoriented, seemed not to understand the question, and growing sadder, stated that he had been depressed many times in his life. The therapist then pointed out that he was not interested in compiling a "diagnostic inventory" but rather in reconstructing this sense of "feeling oneself to be another person," and that the best way to start this was to see if he had felt it on other occasions. After a moment's reflection, Richard noted that a couple of occasions came to mind: the first months after going abroad against the advice of his parents at the age of 19, and immediately after getting married at 31. In both cases he felt as if "turned upside-down," quite different from how he had been feeling shortly before, and he had also felt moments of great desperation and anxiety. However, perhaps because he was younger, he then felt he had "more guts" and will to struggle, and this had allowed him to live through it in a way different from what was happening to him now. Finally—and he pointed this out particularly—they were periods of great suffering which had then turned into big changes in his life. Indeed, after that journey abroad he never returned to the bosom of the family, and acquired an autonomy and an ability to go it alone of which he was still proud. His marriage radically changed his nomadic habits, deeply affecting his private and professional way of life.

The therapist then pointed out how, in effect, the remembered situations seemed to correspond to those "transformations of the sense of self" that commonly appear in the course of individual lifespan development; that it is a characteristic of human experience to feel them as an "overturning of the self" which is always painful, or at least upsetting, because of the need that we have for continuity and integrity; that most of the time we try to avoid these transformations or fight against them because of this need; and that, finally, what he was now feeling could well be the expression of a transformation in progress, since such changes are not associated solely with youth or the first phases of adulthood. Certainly, there were doubtless differences, possibly attributable to the way these changes were experienced, but these differences did not seem to be attributable only to age. Indeed, the main difference seemed to be that while the remembered situations were transformations that had gotten under way following decisions he had made, the present transformation was spontaneous, and it was perhaps because of this that he felt it to be something he had been plunged into involuntarily.

It thus became evident that it was necessary to reconstruct what was changing in him in order to understand and hence be able to do something about the unease it was causing. The only way in which to begin the process of reconstruction was to begin, during the week, to focus on *the form* of the reactions of sudden desperation and the explosions of uncontrollable rage (and not why they were produced), that is, the way in which, day by day, he felt this transformation in progress.

As a last intervention, and so as not to leave out any of the most intense emotional tonalities touched on during the session, the therapist referred to the theme of suicide which Richard had mentioned with a choking voice. He pointed out that the theme of suicide is a possibility that we have in contrast to other animals because of reflexive self-consciousness, and as such belongs to the dimension of human experience itself. It is thus not cause for alarm or shock to feel it at the time when one is feeling particularly intense and perturbing emotions or moods. On the contrary, instead of limiting ourselves to the usual considerations accompanying the surfacing of this theme, it would perhaps be more useful for the work under way to focus on the *how* (which emotions and images precede it and accompany it) and the *when* (in which events and circumstances it appears) of its surfacing. This would allow us to understand if this suicide theme was also one of the ways of feeling the transformation he is undergoing.

Richard's uncommon ability to immediately grasp the new aspects which were emerging, combined with the good emotional and collaborative climate which had been established, made it possible for the reformulation of the problem presented to be completed during the first session.

In Sandra's case the reformulation took about three sessions and schematically followed this course:

The therapist maintained an understanding and tranquilizing attitude while Sandra explained her disturbances; he participated without getting unduly upset in all the situations where she started to cry, and in the end agreed that the most important aspect to be investigated was indeed that of the "fear of losing control," which she had herself brought up several times. First of all, examining with her the events of the last year, the therapist pointed out that this fear did not seem to crop up "at random," in a bizarre and unpredictable manner, but instead seemed to occur within two essential experiential domains: either situations perceived as constrictive (being alone in the car in traffic, feeling it a "duty" to deal with the cooking when her husband and son were present) or situations perceived as leaving her insufficiently protected (being alone at home). Furthermore, while admitting that one was dealing with a disturbing mental state, the therapist nonetheless asked for elucidation on the make-up of this feeling of "losing control" in these situations as if it were the worst thing that could happen to her in her life.

Her responses indicated both the importance attributed to the theme of control as a life value ("being in control is the only way of facing life successfully") and the fact that she exercised continual control over what she felt, even, for example, over physical fatigue, which in her opinion should never go beyond a certain limit or it became alarming. All this was so evident to her that she was not at all surprised to hear that her fear of losing control appeared to be that of a person who, already exercising the maximum possible control over herself, feared the possibility of having to face a further increase. In fact, she maintained that none of this seemed at all strange to her, even though she had never thought of it until now.

The focus shifted, then, to how this need to increase control to maximal levels comes about, and to what makes her feel it to be ever present and necessary. It thus became natural to take up the theme of her mother's death and her ensuing sense of not feeling sufficiently protected. Following rough reconstruction of this most recent period, there emerged the role of her husband in this pervasive sense of nonprotection. The business of the abortion had changed her ideas about what sort of person her husband was. He now seemed totally unreliable, given that he had preferred to lose a child rather than give up some of his comforts. Finally, the superficial and hurried way he behaved on the death of her mother, which followed soon afterwards, dramatically demonstrated for her that she was alone at the mercy of an irresponsible egoist.

All this had gradually permitted an "internal" reformulation of the problem. In comparison with its presentation as an illness, now it was discussed, and she agreed in this, in terms of her emotions and attitudes toward life. Now, finally, through such reformulation it became possible to define a corresponding self-observational setting; this involved both reconstructing the *how* and the *when* of all her perceptions of possible loss of control and also reconstructing the make-up of all the senses of nonprotection which were brought on by the verbal and nonverbal attitudes of her husband, directly observed or inferred.

The trend of the reformulation was not as linear as it may seem, as it was interrupted several times by requests for reassurance as to the possibility of a cure and by more or less explicit attempts by Sandra to divert attention to such themes as illness, medicines, etc. The therapist did not refuse the assurance requested, nor criticize the requests, but tried to use them to advance the process. Hence, while supplying the reassurance requested, the therapist pointed out that these sudden shiftings from talking about her own moods to talking in terms of illness and curability showed a curious extraneous attitude toward her own emotions which would have to be focused on and redefined just as was being done with other aspects of the problem.

With regard to Winnie, reaching a reformulation was a little more laborious, in fact took four or five sessions, and necessitated giving homework right from the initial phase, usually standard practice at the beginning of the second phase. Rather than describing the course of the sessions, it is perhaps more convenient in terms of brevity and conciseness to outline the technical problem the therapist was faced with in working toward a reformulation, and the way used to resolve it.

The procedure for reaching a reformulation in an eating disorders problem varies according to the features of the setting (e.g., ambiguity, reluctance to open up), but the final objective is nearly always more or less the same.

Usually, the problem is presented in terms of an "objective" aesthetic or intellectual unacceptability deriving from a lack of will or cognitive ability, resulting from genetic factors and thus not calling directly into question the person's way of being (external attribution). Without denying or contradicting the problem presented, the therapist must introduce a change of perspective in which the problem seems to consist of how to "cope with others" and, more particularly, in which this difficulty in coping with others depends on one's oversensitivity to their judgments, both anticipated and real. In this manner, as well as reaching an "internal" reformulation, one is also able to define a proper self-observation setting in which to begin the therapy. One begins by focusing on everyday instances of such hypersensitivity in order to gradually proceed with its reconstruction.

The difficulty encountered by the therapist generally involves the emotional-interpersonal context (vagueness, reluctance toward any defined therapeutic commitment, etc.) while, on the other hand, it seems "technically" fairly simple to achieve one's aim. Right from the initial sessions, in fact, such clients behave and talk in such a way that as soon as one reorients their attention, it immediately becomes clear to them that they are prey to the fear of others' judgments.

With Winnie the difficulty was that while from her reports there clearly emerged problems linked to the judgment of others (hypersensitivity to "pressure" put on her by her parents, especially her mother; refusing to "open up" with others of her own age, etc.), it was nevertheless nearly impossible to point them out in her way of being in the session. When faced with requests for elucidation of what she had just said, her level of bewilderment and vagueness was such as to allow her only to repeat, almost mechanically, explanations and opinions long heard in the family. The moment she was asked what she felt in those situations, or what effect they had on her, she became even more bewildered and after a while, with some difficulty, would come up with vague terms like "unease," "discomfort," etc., which she could not even link to people or situations. The only aspect that emerged was that these feelings of unease were more intense at school than at home, even though she was unable to supply any explanation as to why this should be so.

The therapist, then, limited himself to proposing to investigate this apparently strange aspect, asking her to do some simple homework during the week: take a whole page for each school day, divide it in half vertically, and indicate, on the left side, the trend of the intensity of the feeling of unease, and on the right, the progress of scholastic events and activities. This homework was gone over together in subsequent sessions, and analyzed page by page to see if this unease could be linked to events or activities. It immediately became clear that the highest intensity of unease invariably coincided with recreational activities (increase in the possibility of face-to-face interactions with peers) while the lowest levels coincided with moments in which everyone's attention "should" have been concentrated on the lesson or teacher's questions (minimum possibility for face-to-face exchanges). Analyzing more closely, in a later homework report, what this reluctance for face-to-face reactions with peers might be based on, Winnie managed to sketch out a fairly elementary explanation in terms of fear of their judgment, which was enough to be able to carry forward the change in perspective.

As can be seen, the therapist totally excluded the possibility which in a more traditional view would have seemed the most immediate and straightforward: beginning a "dialectical confrontation" with Winnie and so managing to persuade her, in one session if possible, that her real problem was the judgment of others. Firstly, the degree of conviction would be completely aleatory in a client with this level of vagueness and hypersensitivity to the judgment of others (and hence also of the therapist), such that in the end, all would be resolved by a "verbal agreement."

Finally, a change of perspective occurs only insofar as it is the client who brings it about, while attempting to manage the discrepancy he or she is forced to face. In other words, the directivity inherent in the approach we are presenting is purely strategic and does not lead to substituting the client's own understanding processes.

In Gregory's case, finally, the reformulation proceeded fairly linearly and developed over two sessions which would almost seem to be distinguishable as "thesis" and "demonstration." This happens with a certain frequency in obsessive problems, especially if the therapist uses, instead of contrasts, the rational ability and logical rigor of the client.

The moment Gregory finished his exposition, the therapist began by pointing out how from the overall trend there clearly stood out the presence of intense emotions, complex moods, terrifying images, etc. (and Gregory agreed with this), and that if we limited ourselves to the reports of what actually happened, we would find ourselves dealing with "ideas" and "ruminations." In other words, attempting to face difficult situations in life using only ideas and thoughts was like trying to reconstruct a mosaic with only two tiles and no outline to go by.

It was thus necessary to begin focusing on the sequence of images, of emotions, and of thoughts which followed one another in critical moments (self-observational setting), while it appeared likely that feelings and images experienced but not fully recognized by his rational decoding might underlie his current problems ("internal" reformulation).

Gregory followed step by step and most attentively the perspective put forward by the therapist, asking at opportune moments for elucidation. He wanted further explanations of the interrelationships between emotions, images, and thoughts, which he then often used to request reassurances as to the "nonseriousness" of his state, or to reiterate his good feelings for his wife and father-in-law. At the end of the session, he asked what instructions he should follow in order to focus on the critical sequences; in this way, he added, he would be able to better reflect during the week on this method, which seemed at the moment to be convincing, thus putting off until the following session the decision as to whether to commit himself to work of this kind. The following session was that of the "demonstration": he first asked for detailed verification as to how he had applied the instructions over the week, which brought with it supplementary elucidations and reassurances about what we were doing. At last put at ease, he declared that he had decided to undertake this work given that simply "doing the exercises" during the week had made him feel a shade better.

It is interesting to note that, in contrast to succeeding phases, certainly longer and more demanding, during which, however, the therapist may "err" without too serious consequences, being in an already established relationship, these first sessions are critical as they do not allow of any kind of error. Indeed, any error reflects on the very structure of the emotional-relational setting in process of formation, and may thus have quite pervasive effects in time. Analogous to what occurs in the formation of any significant bond, during Phase 1, there are gradually defined—mostly implicitly, as in any affective relationship—the roles and the relational rules that will constrain the structure of the relationship from that moment on.

7

Construing the Therapeutic Setting

This is the central phase of therapeutic strategy, where fairly stable and often complete remission of initial disturbances usually occur. Schematically, it consists of two main phases, each lasting from a minimum of 3 or 4 months to a maximum of 7 or 8, and occurring in succession.

FOCUSING AND REORDERING IMMEDIATE EXPERIENCING

(immediately following the first sessions, up to the 4th–8th month)

The first phase begins with a request from the therapist to put into focus, and later to note down, the events of the week that have been chosen as meaningful on the basis of the reformulation of the initial problem as arrived at in preceding sessions. Analyzing these with the therapist, the client becomes able to break down these events using the sequence of main scenes that make them up, and thus he or she begins the scene-analysis procedure, gradually acquiring the skills essential for managing the self-observation method (e.g., going back and forth in slow motion, zooming in/out). It is essential that from this moment the therapist systematically give self-observational homework for the client to carry out during the week, the analysis of which supplies a starting point for the following session. This is not simply a matter of "keeping a diary," in which it is possible to wander from the point and which often provides rather superficial information. Quite the contrary, clients must be trained to differentiate between various aspects of subjective experiencing until they are able to put one of these aspects into focus and to reconstruct it from various viewpoints. Thus, the usual homework consists of focusing on the specific self-observational item being reconstructed at that moment with the therapist, following its development during the week, and adding further aspects to the reconstruction in progress. Sessions are once a week in order to facilitate clients' more active role in their own self-observation.

During the initial sessions it is absolutely essential that the therapist, using the moviola setting, repeatedly instruct clients to focus, for each scene, on the difference between immediate experiencing and their explaining of it during and after the scene. Introducing the distinction between "how" (experiencing) and "why" (explaining), the therapist should point out that the "how" has to do with subjective experiencing, both in terms of *how it is made up*, that is, its ingredients (e.g., ongoing patterns of flowing imagery; multifaceted, opposing feelings; the felt sense of self) and in terms of *how it comes about*, that is, what *perception* of events or circumstances brought it on.

Thus, for Richard, it was a matter of differentiating his experiencing of helplessness and anger (together with the immediate effect this had on his current sense of self at the moment in which he perceived it) with respect to the conclusions he drew about himself and his life and to the memories of which he immediately became aware. For Sandra, it was a question of focusing on her free-floating experiences of being on the verge of losing control and/or being insufficiently protected, differentiating them from the "logical," "medical," "meteorological" deductions and inferences that she used to explain them. For Winnie, it meant focusing on her pervasive experience of being at the mercy of others' judgments, differentiating it from family expectations of her behavior which she had endorsed. And for Gregory, it meant differentiating his immediately experienced ambivalent feelings and images from the ruminations with which he attempted to explain and control them.

Clients do not acquire this differentiation procedure easily, if for not other reason than the fact that it is so different from their usual manner of living and thinking about their lives. Patience is required to carry on a work of gradual reconstruction and supplying all the explanations necessary, and the therapist should constantly train clients' flexibility in shifting their viewpoint from the "why" to the "how," while reconstructing with them their difficulties in doing so.

Richard, for example, had no "technical" difficulty putting into focus his subjective experiencing; his problem was differentiating helplessness and anger from his subjective experiencing, given that the former seemed to him to be part and parcel of the latter. For Sandra, on the other hand, the difficulties derived from her "sensory reading" of subjective experiencing, so much so that any emotional state was perceived only in terms of neurovegetative reactions (tachycardia, respiratory difficulties, etc.) immediately equated with disease. Winnie's difficulty in focusing on subjective experiencing resulted from her vague and continually oscillating perception of internal states, since thoughts and words seemed to her to be more consistent and reliable. Gregory had difficulty distinguishing thoughts from emotions and ideas from images.

One usually notices that clients begin to be able to put into practice an experiencing/explaining differentiation not only because they apply it more or less correctly in their weekly reports, but also because they gradually begin to extend such differentiation to other experiential domains, so much so that at times it seems to become their usual way of reflecting on things in general. All this is further brought out by a greater capacity to bring critical feelings into focus; this is accompanied, as a rule, by an increased distancing from the immediacy of their experiencing, which further increases the focus. Indeed, this is a suitable point at which to explain to the client that the dynamics of emotional life have various aspects, some stable (background ongoing emotional modulation intertwined with parallel mood oscillations) and others episodic (prominent affective processes matched by intensity peaks). These explanations must be accompanied by adequate instructions to enable them to recognize these aspects and to focus on them.

Furthermore, the ability to differentiate between subjective and objective viewpoints—supported and brought forward in parallel by the therapist—gradually enables the client to see him- or herself from without while experiencing perturbing affects. Clients can thus become aware of attitudes, postures, omitted reactions, etc., which may have escaped a preliminary focusing, and which begin to appear to them in a different light than that which, in the same situation, they had previously thought or imagined.

Richard, for example, began to notice that his uncontrolled outbursts of anger toward others—far from being the expression of his attitude toward living alone, to which he should have resigned himself—instead corresponded to exasperated reactions of protest which went along with equally exasperated perceptions of their emotional detachment. This was particularly evident where his wife was concerned, as he sensed a cooling in their relationship (which for the moment he preferred not to talk about); it was with her that the most intense and uncontrollable outbursts of rage came about.

Looking at her situation from the outside in the focusing of her fear attacks, Sandra began to note with surprise that, rather than being "spontaneous," her fears of losing control were "constructed," so much so that they corresponded to real "tests of strength" to which she deliberately submitted herself; the minute she had a moment's rest, and with nothing in the immediate context to bring it on, she began to imagine vividly everything she feared the most (generally, constricting situations, or being abandoned by her husband) in order to check her capacity for emotional resilience. So if, for example, she reviewed at a glance the reports of several weeks, it immediately became evident that the periods which should have been those of greatest well-being (e.g., when all the family was happily together and her husband was being solicitous toward her) were instead those in which there occurred the highest frequency and intensity of fear attacks. That is not all: they occurred even in situations when, feeling unexpectedly at ease in a feared situation (e.g., alone at home or in the car), she was amazed that she managed "paradoxically" to frighten herself precisely because of having felt at ease. Thus it became gradually clearer to her that her panic attacks were primarily a response to a sort of "internal logic"; that is, they were much more highly correlated to her way of experiencing the relationship with her husband than to his "objective" nonprotective behavior.

Guided step-by-step by the therapist in her subjective/objective shift while focusing on scenes concerning the fear of "not feeling anything anymore" and of the judgment of others, Winnie started to realize that these fears apparently were contrary to what she had maintained; that is, that they were more intense at home than out-side. In situations where she was interacting with those of her same age group, the fear of judgment and of "not feeling" were very intense *immediately before* contact with them, then faded away almost com-pletely, allowing her to relax; these fears, however, were quite low (if not almost absent) when she returned to her family, then *while she spent time at home* they intensified to the point of being so pervasive that they prevented her from engaging in any activity, (e.g., reading, watching television, studying); usually, they reached their highest point on going to sleep, at the time when she seemed to herself so emptied that she felt almost evanescent. Given that at home the pattern of her fears was distinctly correlated not just to the attitudes adopted by her mother, but also simply to her presence, it became clear that our work had to focus more and more on her way of experiencing her relationship with her mother.

For a skeptical Gregory, the unusual opportunity to put into focus feelings and free-floating sequences of images from different points of view revealed that the majority of the "nasty ideas" over which he ruminated were preceded by ambivalent feelings, or feelings of opposition and/or hostility, when he was faced with his father-in-law and/or his wife. Dealing with the former brought him up against the intrusiveness of the man's character, which owed its strength to experience and to professional acumen, and which would inevitably transform Gregory into a docile, undemanding clerk, or even just someone who "knew his place." The hostility toward his wife he explained by saying that she never took sides with him in arguments with his father-in-law. Thus, for example, his ruminations of an evening were much more intense and prolonged, and concerned fairly macabre ideas of illness, if preceded by a disagreement with his father-in-law in which his wife encouraged him to give in, as she usually did, if for no other reason than the respect due to age.

It also became very evident that the hostility and oppositional tendency toward his wife were not entirely traceable to the mere presence of an external factor (e.g., the interference of his father-in-law), as Gregory vigorously maintained. Putting into careful focus all the situations from which this interference could be excluded (when they were alone on holiday or during weekends), it was clear that his ruminations were still present, even though they seemed to follow a slightly different course. Because of his "problems," in fact, their sex life had undergone a progressive "rarefaction" (one may recall his "falling asleep" every evening) of which his wife complained, with the result that he felt she did not understand his suffering; indeed, precisely the fact that his wife was "so interested in sex despite my suffering" was what frequently set off the fear of her possible inclination to prostitution. Ruminations immediately began concerning "remorse toward my wife" which reached the insistent and distressing theme of "I am a wicked man, I have to leave her." At this point, only long, drawn-out reassurances from his wife seemed able to calm him until he "fell asleep" with the usual ritual of tranquilizers and alcohol. It thus became evident for him as well that we were dealing with the presence of, if nothing else, difficulties in managing domains such as sexual intimacy, face-to-face emotional exchanges, etc., none of which surprised Gregory very much, given that he ascribed it wholesale to his rigid religious upbringing.

In any case, while initially the problem had seemed to him to be more "externally bound" and connected with doubts concerning attitudes or concrete decisions to be made (e.g., voicing his own opinion to his father-in-law; changing his job), as the viewpoint-shifting work proceeded, it became clear to him that the problem might be more "internally bound" and concern his way of managing certain immediate aspects of his subjective experiencing. Thus it was that when the therapist proposed shifting the self-observational focus in order to reconstruct both the modality of experiencing anger, hostility, opposition, etc., and also the modality of recognizing and self-referring them, Gregory agreed to what seemed to him a logical, legitimate decision.

At this point, which is generally reached in a range of 1 to 3 months, the client has passed, fairly firmly, from an "externally bound" (putting up with an "objective" problem) to a more "internally bound" attitude (the problem consists of managing one's subjective experiencing). The focus within the "moviola" setting shifts more and more onto the emerging discrepancy between immediate experience and its explicit reordering, with the agreed objective of reconstructing the actual pattern of coherence on which it depends.

It thus becomes possible, on the one hand, to further widen the focus on perturbing feelings, reconstructing their various links with other aspects of immediate experience, making the client progressively realize how any emotional state—besides being multifaceted

and including the experience of opposing feelings—is always a construction that entails processes of recognition and self-referring. On
the other hand, in reconstructing the client's way of elaborating
beliefs and expectations out of ongoing immediate experience, the
boundaries begin to emerge of his or her current self-image and the
self-deceiving patterns for maintaining it. We are here dealing with
the remaining work of this first stage, which essentially consists of
reconstructing the client's current pattern of coherence and the ways
in which its imbalance gives rise to the original problems.

With the work done so far, Richard had reached a good level of
focusing and distancing on his helplessness/anger outbursts, to the
point where they afflicted him far less and had become less frequent
and less intense. The situation with his wife appeared little changed,
however, if not worse. The alternation of outbursts of uncontrolled
anger with desperate reactions of "abandonment" had become even
more intense and repetitive. Despite the reluctance he had always
shown in talking about it, he agreed, through the force of circumstances, to put his experiencing of the actual interactions and exchanges with his wife in the "moviola" setting.

Shifting continuously from subjective to objective viewpoint, it
became fairly clear that his outbursts of rage were replete with grudges
and accusations against her, and that these were set off whenever he
interpreted an attitude of his wife's in terms of sexual refusal. Within,
generally, a very short space of time, an abandoning reaction would
emerge, in which he felt he did not deserve his wife, leading to a kind
of ataraxic indifference, in which he would not have batted an eyelid
even if his wife had suddenly announced that she wanted a divorce.
Richard was astonished to discover that his outbursts of anger were
prevalently made up of "sexual grudges" toward his wife, given that
(and he seemed at last to have conquered his reluctance to talk about
the matter) he himself had decided more than 2 years previously to
cease any kind of sexual activity with his wife. In putting into focus
how this decision had come about, what seemed to be the critical
event emerged.

About 3 years previously, on an evening apparently like any
other, his wife had heedlessly let slip that she had had an affair with
one of her colleagues whom he knew only by sight. At the moment of
this revelation, Richard was stunned, but immediately afterwards he
exploded into such a violent rage that his wife considered calling the

police. He suddenly calmed down, took his wife into the bedroom, and in a peremptory, contemptuous fashion forced her to give "technical" demonstrations of all the erotic situations (including her own contribution) that had come about during every single meeting with the other. While his intention had been to profoundly humiliate her, he unexpectedly found himself victim of a sexual excitement he had never known before. He thus "couldn't help" transforming all of this into a procedure repeated every night on going to bed. Naturally, after this had gone on for a few weeks, his wife burst into tears threatening divorce because of "sexual incompatibility" due to his obvious perversion. This led, however, to a reversal of the situation, with his wife attributing her extramarital affair to his sexual "oddity" which she had always intuited, and which had finally come to light. Richard, meanwhile, became more and more convinced that he was despicable and shamefully perverted, and announced that he was willing to give up all sexual activity between them and to allow his wife sexual freedom as long as she withdrew her threat of divorce.

Several sessions were needed in order to accurately "run through the moviola" his experiencing of the whole event using the scene-analysis procedure and the subjective/objective shifting method with which he was by now well acquainted. A picture gradually emerged which was quite different from that which Richard had built up for himself in the course of these 3 years.

While he felt stunned and, gradually, while he was prey to unrestrained fury, she had lost in his eyes that image of "innocent child," "poetically ingenuous" (she was 12 years younger than he), which only he could have preserved intact in time, in the face of an external reality that is quite indifferent to such sentiments. Only when he could see her rendered submissive and humiliated by his oppression did he realize that his wife was still, after all, "his baby"; however, he had shown himself to be a "bad father," quite incapable of protecting her from the perils of the world. At the point when his wife burst into tears and threatened divorce, this reversal procedure reached its height. Richard, who felt himself "no longer worthy of her," was ready to do anything to stay living together, although he did not deserve it. In other words, the connecting thread in his way of experiencing the whole situation was represented by the unexpected alteration of the image of his wife, triggered at the moment of the revelation, and of the succeeding modalities with which he sought to erase and/or negate the perceived change. The "sexual perversions" were hence seen as a basic self-deceiving pattern which, radically altering in a negative sense his own self-image, made the image of his wife, by contrast, appear positive once more.

It should be pointed out that during the session in which all of this became clear to him, Richard underwent a strong emotional reaction: he was extremely moved and quite unable to hold back his tears, saying again and again that as an undoubted "monster," he could never have imagined being someone who would throw blame on himself in order to preserve the image of a loved one. With the benefit of hindsight in looking back over the progress of the therapy, one can safely say that this was one of the "key" sessions of the process, giving rise to a significant change in his behavior, which became less resigned, less desperately fixed in the role of one "abandoned for life," and more enterprising in carrying on the exploratory work that had "awakened" him.

Finally, "running everything through the moviola" from then until now, it was evident to him that the expectation of a *coup de théâtre* in which his wife would come back to him, ready to accept even his "perversion" (which, among other things, had vanished upon the threat of divorce), had never left him, but had instead functioned as a steady background from which he could project a possible future. He had in fact discovered that the times of blackest desperation, when he thought of suicide, always corresponded to those afternoons when he "intuited" that his wife was meeting her current boyfriend, and the resulting outbursts of anger invariably occurred when she came home from the supposed meeting.

Sandra's greater ability to focus on perturbing feelings while shifting the viewpoint onto herself went along with a greater ability to recognize in the ongoing emotional states other aspects beyond the purely "sensory" and with an increased ability in distancing from the immediacy of her fears.

This made her realize that her panic attacks, rather than being simply a more or less automatic response to situations perceived by her as constrictive (being alone in the car in the midst of traffic) or nonprotective (being alone at home), were a continual "showing herself" that instead of being the strong woman capable of controlling herself that she should have been, she was instead one who could lose control at any moment, and this required the presence of a reference figure to "keep an eye on her," this figure being her husband. It also put her in a position to be able to begin reconstructing the multi-faceted aspects with which she was experiencing the marital relation-ship; such an undertaking would have been arduous, to say the least, in preceding sessions, where she expressed herself almost exclusively in terms of tachycardia, dyspnea, high blood pressure, etc., and the only emotional state she seemed able to recognize was fear.

And so she agreed to begin the reconstruction by starting from the "disappointments" with her husband which had first appeared about a year and a half previously, and only fleetingly referred to in preceding sessions. The critical events for her which were to be "run through the moviola" with great accuracy were roughly as follows.

When her husband urged an abortion, or when he showed an unusual hurry at her mother's funeral, it did not strike her as being very important, and she attributed it to the "male selfishness" her mother had often told her about. Indeed, it was an indirect confirma-tion that her husband, who paid little attention to "feminine sensitiv-ity," was in fact the strong, virile decisive man she had always desired. The important event came about a month before the first panic attack, when quite by chance she found out that her husband had several times boasted of being able to dominate his passions as few other men could, having emerged unscathed some months previously from a tumultuous sexual affair that would have overwhelmed anyone else. Sandra immediately attributed his behavior over the abortion and the funeral to the fact that he was completely taken up by this affair. She felt her "pride was hurt," and that she was "challenged" by her husband's arrogance, so much so that a month later, in order to spite him, she had an affair with his best friend, whom she had long found attractive. The meeting turned out to be particularly exciting for her, to the point where she felt pleasurably perturbed. Perhaps because of this perturbation, she began to think, while returning home, that it would not be a good idea to continue this challenge with her husband, as she would certainly be less able than he to control herself, and might end up doing something stupid (like running away with someone else) which for the rest of her life she would have to pay for. It was in that moment that she had her first panic attack.

Going back and forth on reconstructed sequences of affect-laden scenes according to the shifting procedure required several sessions (eight to ten), and eventually these scenes began to take on another appearance.

Hence, in repeatedly running through the "moviola" the scene where she first heard about her husband's affair, it became clear to her that it was not the "sexual betrayal" that had disillusioned her as much as the fact that her husband had boasted of it to his friends; if while observing herself from without she put this aspect particularly into focus, it was clear that this "arrogance" of her husband's made him look like an "adolescent seeking approval from his peer group." Having always viewed her husband as an adult *par excellence,* she was astonished by this new perception. It also enabled her to relate it to her husband's way of doing other things, which she now saw in quite a different light. His way of working was an example. The fact that her husband continually changed his work plans, setting off on the most disparate undertakings, often going from one sector to another diametrically opposite, was for her an overpowering example of his unshakable autonomy and initiative. Now, however, she began to see that her husband had still not decided "what to do when he grew up," and in the meantime the only guaranteed salary was that from her own work. What astonished her most, as she dwelt on this aspect, was that this was only clear to her now, while it was something that she was certain she had experienced at the moment of that fateful revelation.

Going on to analyze the scenes regarding her affair with her husband's friend, it became clear that the spite motive had played an absolutely secondary role in the whole business. She had always felt an intense reciprocal attraction for this man, who was independent, sure of himself, and had attained considerable professional success. More than once she had indulged in unrestrained fantasies, and only the certainty that she was married to a man who was his superior "by strength of character" had made her regard them as romantic fancies. The perturbation she had felt during their meeting was equated by her with the unexpected and unpleasant realization that, while her husband made himself look good in front of his friends but invariably returned to the roost, for her there was the "real" possibility of never going back again. Suddenly seeing the home broken up and her husband abandoned presented her with an absolutely unacceptable picture of herself. In the female role model she had borrowed from her mother, who all her life had put up with Sandra's often violent and drunken father, self-sacrifice in the cause of family unity played a central role, and only a "crazy" or "irresponsible" woman would think of endangering it. Therefore it began to be increasingly clear that the exclusion from consciousness of the feelings inherent either in the

perceived change in the husband's image or in the emotional involvement experienced had become the essential self-deceiving mechanism
for maintaining her usual sense of self. In the final analysis, this made
even more evident the paradoxical aspect of the situation, in which
the excluded feelings could only be appraised and recognized as uncontrollable fears of being alone or losing control, which by limiting
her autonomy forced her to search for closer contact with a partner
whom she would otherwise feel she had every right to leave. It was just
this paradoxical aspect that led her to the behavior toward her husband which at first sight seemed strange and contradictory. On the
one hand, the minimum physical separation from him seemed absolutely intolerable for her, and, on the other, the moment he was
present, any contact with him seemed equally intolerable, and she felt
ever more constricted and irritable until she was afraid she could no
longer control herself.

While training Winnie in the "moviola" setting for reconstructing affect-laden scenes, the therapist took particular care to foster her
ability to recognize and appraise ongoing feelings and emotional states
and also gradually to focus her attention on the role played in her
unease by her fear of judgment by others (an particularly by her
mother). More than ten sessions were needed for her perception of
her internal states to become less fluctuating and uncertain, and to
lead her to a position where she was able to put into focus the emotions she felt in given moments and to refer them back to what had
triggered them. Only when she seemed less lost and reluctant to
open up was it possible to begin reconstructing one aspect that from
the beginning had seemed critical for her, that is, her experiencing
of her relationship with her mother. The main stages marking
this process of reconstruction and reordering may be outlined as
follows.

During the process of breaking down the trend of the unease she
felt at home into the corresponding critical scenes, it emerged that the
greatest intensity of anxiety invariably corresponded either to situations in which Winnie perceived her mother's attitudes and opinions
as negative judgments or to situations in which, anticipating such
attitudes or opinions, Winnie felt she did not live up to her mother's
expectations of her. Hence, for example, the growing level of anxiety while going to sleep was due to her monitoring what she had
done during the day from her mother's point of view, feeling more and

more inadequate and incompetent. At this point it was clear even to her that this continual referral to possible expectations on the part of her mother in order to anticipate any possible negative judgments was substantially the basic regulator of her day.

Once she had reached the point of being able to recognize these situations with some ease, the critical scenes were put into still sharper focus, guiding her in observing herself both from within the scene and from without, while going back and forth in slow motion. In this way it became progressively more evident to her that in perceiving a negative judgment, or feeling that she did not match up to expectations, the critical element was that Winnie *immediately* imagined the possible picture her mother had of her. If after dinner, for example, her mother, commenting with others on what they had seen on television recently, alluded, even faintly, to the theme of the ingratitude of children, Winnie immediately felt that her mother saw her as an egoist, incapable of genuine sentiments, and thus, in the end, ungrateful.

Putting into sharper focus, in the "moviola" setting, the *moment* in which she imagined her mother's image of her, it slowly grew clearer to her how the perception of that image became part of the sense of self that she felt at that moment. In other words, as soon as she saw herself as ungrateful in her mother's eyes, she immediately *experienced* herself as ungrateful. Hence Winnie was carefully trained to capture this shifting—"how the perception of another's attitude corresponded to the definition of a sense of self"—not only with her mother (where the process took on obvious and recognizable forms), but also with anyone else toward whom she felt even the minimum fear of judgment. Until Winnie was able to grasp this aspect even in situations which she took to be negligible, the therapist felt it would not be wise to pass onto the next phase.

At this point, the therapist began the structuring of a self-observational setting which would increase her flexibility with others' perspective taking and would foster a modification of the viewpoint on herself *concomitant* with a modification of her way of seeing others. The rationale for the new procedure being undertaken was clearly and concisely outlined. It was explained, in simple terms, that the behavior of others consisted substantially of information, and that this could be read or codified either as information about oneself or as information about others; that in the first case, one tries to draw an image of oneself from others, taking no account of whom they may be, while in the second case, one tries to see how others might be, independently of we who are looking at them.

Thus, the simplest way of carrying on this new differentiation consisted of putting into focus, "in the moviola," a critical attitude perceived in another, and so to begin to train oneself, with the therapist's help, to shift from one to the other viewpoint, following this scheme:

	S —	PERCEIVING A'S BEHAVIOR AS INFORMATION ABOUT
	H	ONESELF
FOCUSING ON	I	(e.g., If A behaves that way, what about me?)
A'S BEHAVIOR	F	
	T	
	I —	PERCEIVING A'S BEHAVIOR AS INFORMATION ABOUT
	N	HIM OR HER
	G	(e.g., If A behaves that way, what about him or her?)

In this way, it became possible for Winnie to differentiate her sense of self from her mother's behavior, searching in this behavior for data which might give her an image of her mother as a person. For example, the victimizing attitudes habitual of her mother which previously brought out in her only an immediate feeling of inadequacy, now began to be seen as "relational modes" with which her mother controlled the members of the family.

While this trend of increasing her flexibility with others' perspective taking was retained for the rest of the therapy, Winnie was now in a position to reconstruct, together with the therapist, how disturbing the unbalancing of her perception of her mother (which was at the origin of the disturbances) could be.

The critical events to be broken down in their corresponding scenes were more or less hinted at in preceding sessions, and, in rapid succession, were as follows.

Her summer flirtation of 10 months previously had been a timid debut into love, and had ended in what was for her a "total defeat." Although her mother had been completely opposed to the idea, the boy was very important to Winnie, and even with her fear of "not feeling enough," she would have been ready to fight to keep it going if she had not realized at a certain point that he did not like her enough. She consequently explained her anorexic reaction as a desperate attempt to fit in with his aesthetic tastes. The failure of this attempt had given her a profound sense of defeat that had "flattened" and "emptied" her, and all this came out at school where she started getting lower marks than usual. Her mother's immediate comment, that "since my daughter lost her head over a good-for-nothing she become such a moron she can't even study," was for Winnie a sudden revelation of incontestable truth, so much so that leaving school was the only way to avoid the humiliation of certain defeat.

Each scene was repeatedly "run through the moviola," constantly maintaining, on the one hand, the differentiation between her sense of self and her mother's behavior, and guiding her, on the other hand, in alternating positions between who is living the scene in person (subjective viewpoint) and who is watching the scene from without (objective viewpoint). It was thus possible to arrive at this kind of reordering.

At the moment of greatest friction during this flirtation, Winnie's mother had applied such intense and theatrical pressure that suddenly Winnie, for the first time in her life, had begun to doubt whether her mother could be the "special woman" she had always believed her to be. If from this moment on one accurately focused on the effect that this unexpected modification of her mother's image had on her, one immediately noticed that the sense of possibly being ugly and fat started to come to the surface at just that time, while in the past it had never occurred to her. It was thus clear to her as well that calling into question, if only for a moment, the positiveness of her image of her mother had immediately triggered a blurred and wavering experiencing of herself appraised as a sense of emptiness and as a fear of not feeling emotions sufficiently. The anorexic reaction, then, turned out to be the self-deceiving mechanism for dropping the boy and putting her mother back into her habitual role, even though this led to being even more "externally bound" to her mother's expectations and judgments in order to define a reliable sense of self. At this point, it was an almost immediate reaction to feel herself unable to carry on the school year the moment she heard her mother put in doubt her learning capabilities and scholastic ability.

The increased ability that Gregory was gradually acquiring in putting into focus his "nasty ideas" while shifting the viewpoint on himself went in parallel with a greater ability to differentiate between immediate experiencing (e.g., uncontrollable feelings, images suddenly coming to the surface intermingled with ambivalent feelings) and attempts to reorder that experience "rationally" (e.g., ruminations, rituals). Indeed, most of the time he managed to put into focus the initial blend of intrusive images and perturbing feelings which had set off the whole sequence of ruminations and rituals, and this had noticeably increased his ability to distance himself from the immediacy of his frightening "insights" and recurrent fears.

In comparison with the first sessions when he concentrated exclusively on the logical thread of his ruminations, Gregory was now able, in the scene-analysis procedure, to put much more accurately into focus both the way he experienced the beginnings of his intolerance over his marital situation, and also his search for some impossible consistency with a self-image that would admit of not even the slightest "shadow" or imperfection. Indeed, if he accepted his intolerance, he immediately felt "wicked" (and this meant he would have to leave his wife). If, on the other hand, he assumed that such intolerance was unfounded he immediately reassured himself as to his presumed wickedness, but felt "impotent" before his tormenting fears. At the "moviola" setting, it came into clear focus that the "effective memory" of scenes in which his wife seemed to be unequivocally on his father-in-law's side was called into question in terms of its "real" validity, with the result that the discrimination "I am wicked"/"I feel impotent" became even more insoluble. And so it became ever clearer to him how the difficulty in self-referring certain aspects of subjective experiences lay in the fact that these experiences, if recognized and appraised, transformed themselves immediately into intolerable doubts about himself.

Running all the scenes thus far analyzed "through the moviola," the work began of reconstructing his rigid all-or-none procedures for maintaining consistency, both in the appraisal of immediate experiencing and in the structuring of an acceptable self-image. Scene by scene, the focus was directed to his way of dichotomizing subjective experiencing into opposing and irreconcilable parts and combining them in such a way that if there was the slightest doubt about one of them (positive self) then the other automatically became true ("wicked self"). A long time had to be spent on this aspect, putting into focus at the "moviola" a wide variety of instances of "all-or-nothing" procedures which, even if they appeared to be negligible, turned out to be extremely useful in increasing his flexibility in experiencing and self-referring.

At this point Gregory had acquired a good command of focusing on his emotional states, distinguishing their opposing and antithetical feelings, and an appreciable flexibility in self-referring them, to the point where "feeling angry" no longer necessarily implied "feeling wicked." Indeed, "new situations" made their appearance, such as those where he got "openly" angry with his wife or father-in-law, something which up to now he had scrupulously avoided. Shortly afterwards, he was amazed to note that at the times in which he got openly angry with his wife because of his father-in-law, he no longer had the usual sequence of nasty ideas and macabre images. His first-hand experience of the "rightness" of the work he had so far carried out was an intense emotional experience which gave rise to moments of exaltation of which he himself, usually so calm and composed, was the first to wonder at. This key session worked as a catalyst on all the work done until that point, and began a consistent change in attitude toward his original problems, which were now directly referred to his way of experiencing his relationship with his wife.

We went on to reconstruct the "unbalancing" in such ex-periencing which had been capable of triggering those ambivalent and perturbing feelings that had involved him in painful ruminations in the course of the last 7 or 8 months. The critical events, which were broken down into their relative scenes in order to be put into focus, turned out to be two, and were as follows:

The first had been about a year previously, at the time of his marriage. During the engagement, Gregory had been tormented by doubts about the advisability of getting married, with the result that he was always putting off the date. As soon as the date had finally been fixed, the doubts became concerned with fitting together all the disparate details of the wedding ceremony, to the point where a couple of days before the wedding he asked his wife for a further postpone-ment for perfectly negligible reasons. His wife, with the irritable tone of one on the verge of tears, reacted in a way that would admit of no reply: "By now I don't care anymore if you don't want to get married," she said, "but I have no intention of making a fool of my father when he has absolutely nothing to do with it. That means we're going to get married on the date we've arranged and then if necessary get divorced straight afterwards." This totally unexpected reply left Gregory rigid, and he was immediately assailed by remorse for having humiliated and offended his wife in what should have been a moment of joy and happiness for her. During the first 4 or 5 months of marriage, this "remorse" gradually increased, both because of the now evident sexual problems and because of the interference of his father-in-law for whom he had started to work immediately after the marriage. One evening after dinner, when Gregory had begun to complain to his wife about the latest humiliation suffered at the hands of his father-in-law, she cut him short with the same irritated tone as before, and said that the fact that he did not get on with her father made their relationship one of simply living together instead of a true marriage. Gregory was once more thunderstruck and remorseful, not fully understanding what his wife meant. Soon afterwards, while going to bed, there suddenly came to mind the image of his father-in-law dangling from the table of a morgue.

Repeatedly running each scene "through the moviola," and using as leverage both his ability to differentiate between immediate experiencing and explicit restructuring, and also his ability to reconstruct all the aspects of a given subjective experience, observing himself alternately from the inside and from the outside of the scenes, we were able to achieve the following reordering:

For the whole period of the engagement, Gregory had severe doubts about the quality and consistency of his own involvement. He was unsure whether it would last a lifetime, and this made him feel that he was in, for him, the untenable position of one who endangers the life of another for what might turn out to be just a whim. It was his wife's behavior, that of total loving and dedication, that calmed his fears and persuaded him that his would surely be a good, positive marriage. A few days before the wedding, at the moment when he had felt himself go rigid at his wife's reply, Gregory had the frightening insight that his wife's loving behavior was neither felt nor spontaneous, but was part of a game of family opportunity, for which his father-in-law wrote the rules. As was already clear to him, accepting that insight and verifying it would have meant, in his all-or-none logic, an unacceptable self-image. The self-deceptive mechanism for trying to maintain the current sense of self thus consisted of denying the reliability of what had been experienced, which in this way became a tormenting fear he had to fight against, but which was foreign to his "real" mode of being.

The event some months later fully confirmed the previous insight, making him feel at the mercy of an unloving wife who took her orders from a tyrannical father-in-law. Nevertheless, the hostility, anger, and disappointment that were thus triggered while, on the one hand, taking direct form by the avoidance of sexuality and the rituals he exasperated his wife with, could, on the other, only be deceptively self-referred as foreign ideas which suddenly dropped into his head.

At this point, usually reached in a period of a minimum of 4 months to a maximum of 8 from the beginning of the therapy, the clients have gone through an appreciable change in their current viewpoint on themselves, accompanied by a remarkable remission of the disturbances which led them to therapy.

At this level, the change basically consists of a shifting from experiencing personal "properties" (disturbances, diseases, somatic complaints, etc.) and "traits" (fear, anger, helplessness, etc.) as constitutionally "given," to appraising them as the living, ongoing dynamics of attributing one's own meanings to things (i.e., through the ability of self-observing one's ways of identifying and ordering meaningful events, of maintaining one's self image, of structuring affective relationships). This shifting of the client's point of view on him- or herself brings about a reordering of immediate experiencing matched by a *first level* of restructuring of the range of perceivable emotions; he or she can recognize and self-refer feelings that were previously neglected or excluded from consciousness, as well as being able to experience many nuances in the same feeling tonality.

Above all, the client is now able to focus on more complex emotional states and to perceive the connection between different feelings and affects, such as the concurrent relationships between attachment, fear, and anger. As we have been able to see, in fact, in the course of the work done in this part, one meets an "implicit" reformulation of the original problem, in the sense that clients become progressively more able to realize and reconstruct how current critical emotional states are interwoven with a perceived imbalance in an affective relationship experienced as essential to their present life structure.

The second part therefore starts out by putting into focus the reformulation reached, and making it explicit in terms of the client's self-referent organization, that is, in which way patterns of personal meaning allow the structuring of affectional ties capable of maintaining the perceived coherence of one's current sense of self. Further widening the focus of exploration and comprehension in the self-observational setting, one thus begins to analyze the client's "affectional style," reconstructing with him or her the recurrent patterns underlying its unity and continuity.

THE RECONSTRUCTION OF THE CLIENT'S AFFECTIVE STYLE

(lasting from 3 to 7 months, i.e., from the 4th–8th month to the 7th–15th month of therapy)

As we have already seen in the discussion of our clients, the essential affective imbalance capable of triggering emotional disturbances usually coincides with a rather abrupt change in the image of the significant figure, whether this is the result of events lived through (disappointments, unforeseen revelations, etc.) or of a mutation of perspective within the client as a result of his or her personal growth (as is the case, for example, with Winnie).

Indeed, the structured image of an attachment figure, through the intermodal coordination of sensory-motor-affective modules, brings about a quality of immediate experiencing ("I") specifically appraised and recognized as one's "real" self ("Me"). In this sense, the change perceived in a significant other's image is matched by a specific "I"/"Me" discrepancy: on the one hand, the experienced interruption in one's ongoing patterns of immediate experience is paralleled by a distressing psychophysiological modulation perceived as an unbearable challenge to one's conscious sense of self; on the other hand, through restricted and distorted explicit reordering processes (exclusion, self-deception, etc.) distressing feelings can be appraised and attibuted to external causes without calling into question the coherence of the self-image thus far structured.

At this juncture, the therapist should make explicit the reformulation of the original problem which has taken place implicitly during the work done up to now, highlighting the correlation between perceived imbalance and the change in the partner's image. Further reconstruction through the "moviola" of the chronological trend of the emergence of the perturbations makes the client realize that the surfacing of perturbing feelings is in parallel with the change in the perception of the partner. Thus, while it becomes more and more apparent that the original problem coincides with the exclusion and the self-deceptive reordering of challenging feelings triggered by a major affective oscillation, it is also necessary to shift the focus onto how the client constructs the image of an attachment figure consistent with the sense of self, and with which mechanisms he or she tries to cope with any discrepancies that may occur. Deepening the self-observation method and reconstructing the self-referent organization exhibited by clients in structuring their affectional bonds thus become the only ways to reconstruct and reorder such mechanisms.

The reconstruction of affective style takes up the entire second part and begins with a detailed analysis of the client's affective history conducted by successively developing the following aspects:

1. Variables (developmental context, personal attitudes, social network) that underlay the "sentimental debut" and the ways in which it was experienced, appraised, and self-referred. The importance of the sentimental debut derives from the fact that it corresponds to a kind of "dress rehearsal" of the career in loving which is just beginning. The ways in which this rehearsal is carried on permits a glimpse at the set of basic ingredients which will be part of the affective style; in addition, the perceived outcome of the rehearsal in the client's eyes, will influence the way in which those ingredients will recombine to give rise to a more specific and defined affective style.

2. The sequence of meaningful relationships that have taken place since the debut, enabling the client to reconstruct the criteria of significance through which he or she is able to differentiate between meaningful and nonmeaningful relationships. Such criteria permit us to highlight which patterns of assortative mating turn out to be most consistent with the bonding style which has been gradually structured.

3. The way in which each meaningful relationship was formed, maintained, and broken, and the ways in which they were experienced, appraised, and self-referred. In this way, it is possible to reveal the coherence exhibited by the client's affective style, that is, how this style is able to produce recurrent emotional experiences which can stabilize and sometimes also further develop his or her current sense of self.

The sequences of significant scenes characterizing each relationship are then repeatedly "passed through the moviola," working with the client's ability both to differentiate between immediate experiencing and explicit restructuring, and to reconstruct the different aspects of a given subjective experience, observing him- or herself alternately from inside and from outside the scene.

The affect-laden events that characterized Richard's affective history—reconstructed by developing the above points—were distributed roughly as follows:

His first love affair occurred when he was about 17, during a period in which, dedicated to the literature and study of cinema, he led a solitary life apart from his fellows, who nicknamed him "the brown bear" not only because of his solitary habits, but also because of his very black, very thick hair. She, a little older, spent a lot of her time with the peer group. He had indulged in unbridled fantasies about her but never showed anything openly, indeed was somewhat bashful, especially in her presence. It was she, her curiosity aroused by his air of being "different" and "intellectual," who took the initiative of being around him more, and then, without much in the way of preamble and to his amazement, asked him directly if they could "start dating." Richard's disbelief transformed almost immediately into a feeling of elation matched by a sense of being exclusively chosen—a feeling he could barely hide, making himself look even more awkward and clumsy. This state of exaltation, however, lasted a very short time, as it soon seemed impossible that this could have really happened to him, and he immediately closed himself up again in his usual retiring, detached manner. The affair lasted only a week, as he found it hard to tolerate her ironic little comments about his being a "bear" or "clumsy," and disliked seeing her enjoying herself with her friends, something which he felt she did not do with him. And so, one afternoon, Richard suddenly had an outburst of uncontrollable rage for some neglible reason he could not even remember, with the result that she went off and never talked to him again, just giving him a nod whenever they happened to meet. Richard had a very intense and prolonged depressive reaction which kept him for months shut up in his room almost in a stupor. After nearly a year, he slowly began to feel the desire to start doing something again, and in order not to end up in the same environment which had caused so much "trouble," he decided to go abroad, despite the opposition of his parents.

After leaving home, Richard led a somewhat adventurous life which gave him the opportunity to have relationships with many women, even though, he reported, after the experience of his first love, he always had difficulty in effectively involving himself in an affair. There were two relationships he indicated as being meaningful: the first lasted from the age of 25 to 29, and the second was with his wife, which started when he was 32. The criteria which permitted the identification of these two relationships as significant were basically reducible to two: having the feeling of being unconditionally chosen by the partner, and feeling a sense of total reliability on the part of the other, deriving from the fact that the latter had left what appeared to be a more advantageous life style in order to be with him.

At the age of 25 he was living abroad, where, after finishing a course in film directing, he had begun working professionally with some success; it was what he called the "best moment of my life," in which he felt he was the leader of his working group and felt he shone in social situations, where he was also much sought after, even though he still had a tendency to lead a rather retiring existence. The affair with this woman, 2 years older than he and from a fairly well-to-do and well-known family, started in a decidedly passionate manner when, during what seemed like a banal flirtation, she suddenly decided to leave her family and live with him. Richard accepted the situation as a *fait accompli*, with little enthusiasm, maintaining that it was impossible and destined to vanish like a soap bubble in a short space of time. Little by little, however, his habits changed, and he dedicated less and less time to work and study, reaching the point where this relationship became the central element of his life structure, even though he appraised all this as just "responding to elementary good manners imposed by living with another person." For a couple of years this situation continued, Richard living it as if under a spell; he appraised every moment as if it marked the end, only to realize a moment later that there was further confirmation that he was her choice, from the way she fought back against the pressure from her family, who had decided at all costs to make her break off this affair. At the end of the second year the situation suddenly cooled; she became vague and elusive, held her own less and less against her family, and after a short space of time packed her bags and went back to them. For some days, Richard suffered deep depression, when all of a sudden he realized, as if the spell had finally broken, that it was precisely his passive attitude, that of being "condemned and awaiting the verdict," which had caused her to leave. He then started a desperate chase that lasted for 2 years, continually running after her and blaming himself for anything and everything if only they could start again, and which finished only when he received a definitive warning from the family lawyer.

The beginning of his love affair with his wife at the age of 32 happened in a different evolutionary context. Richard returned for good to his own country, where he made a brilliant start as a television director. The outcome of his previous affair increased his difficulty in involving himself in further relationships, and emphasized the futility of overwhelming intense affairs, bringing about the feeling that his life as a bachelor was coming to an end and that he "had to get his head together." His future wife, who was 12 years younger than he, was one of his students, who, after being in a state of ecstatic adoration for about a year, finally decided to ask him if there was any chance of their getting together. Richard did not consider it an obstacle that he felt neither passion nor enthusiasm; indeed it looked to him like a situation offered by fate to enable him to start living just like everybody else. During the first year of marriage, however, he felt progressively more disappointed by his wife, whose immediacy and ingenuousness began to look more and more like immaturity. When she became pregnant, he went into an intense depressive crisis, which, as had emerged in the first sessions, was characterized by a disturbing sense of "feeling like another person." He came out of it with the perspective that from that moment on, his life must be centered on his wife and child, that is, on his "two children," as if to say that he had changed from being a bachelor to being a widower with two children. As a consequence he changed his life commitment, putting his career as television director, which had been his only objective, into second place.

Repeatedly "passing through the moviola" the reconstructed sequence of critical events on the basis of the by now well-established scene-analysis procedure, the essential ingredients on which the self-organization of his affective style was based became clear to him.

In the first place, the centrality of the experience of loss leapt into view as the connecting theme running through his whole way of structuring affective relationships. Thus, the anticipated perception of loss appeared as the ordering element of how a relationship was started, as emerges from the first experience (it seeming impossible that this should actually be happening to him), and the affair started at age 25 (his feeling that her decision was a "soap bubble"), and also his relationship with his wife, in which the "absence" of emotional reciprocity (lack of enthusiasm and passion) had been the very condition permitting the formation of the relationship. The explicit requisite of perceiving himself as the "object of choice" on the part of the partner emphasized, furthermore, that Richard felt it was he himself who was the "cause" of this impending loss ("internal" causal attribution). It was precisely his pervasive sense of unlovableness which led him to categorically exclude the possibility of taking the initiative in any courting situation, even when he felt that there was mutual attraction.

The trend of each relationship proceeded in a manner similar to its inception; here too, in fact, the continuous anticipation of loss seemed to give him a key for reading the trend of things ("made fun of and mistreated" in his first experience, "condemned and awaiting the verdict" at 25, "widower" in his marriage), confirming and stabilizing his ongoing sense of being-in-the-world (that of being alone, abandoned, inexorably separated from life and others). At the same time, his minimizing of the life changes that accompanied his relationships by attributing them to external factors such as "good manners" or the "childishness" of his wife corresponded to a systematic failure to acknowledge, through self-deceptive mechanisms, the range and intensity of his own emotional involvement; besides, in a world in which loss is experienced as certain and inevitable, "not being attached to anybody" could not but appear to him as the most effective way of reducing the intensity of disruptive feelings from detachments, rejections, and so on, which he assumed must regularly occur.

Finally, the experience of loss unmistakably marked all the crises and break-ups of his affective relationships. In the first place, it was invariably the partner who took the initiative to end it, and Richard passively "suffered" an abandonment which to him was the definitive confirmation of what he had always felt, despite the fact that he had more than once realized how he himself had brought about this abandonment (the outburst of rage on the first occasion, the passive attitude held during the cohabitation started when he was 25, treating his wife from the start as a "retarded child"). Once the break-up had happened, the excessive increase of the sense of his own negativity and unlovableness was the only way to recover a more active role, supplying an explanation of what had happened which would be sufficiently consistent for him, and would at the same time allow him to struggle to recover what had been lost. The episode of "sexual perversion" with his wife, which had played an important part in the first part of the work, was where this attitude stood out most clearly.

In Sandra's case, the critical events of her affective history, reconstructed by developing in succession the usual points, gave rise to the following profile:

Her debut occurred when she was around 16–17, in the midst of various difficulties deriving from the familial developmental context. Her father, besides being emotionally absent from the family, exercised firm control over his daughter, as if she were some kind of inept fool quite incapable of taking care of herself and thus prey to any man who happened to pass by. It was therefore almost impossible to go out when she had time off from studying; parties were forbidden, as were trips or any other occasion for spending time with her peers. The only friends admitted to the house were the few young women who had passed through the screening examination of her father. Her mother, even though not agreeing with her husband, whose continual irascibility and violence she had to suffer, was nonetheless relieved that Sandra was safe from the perils of the world and from the traps laid by men, which she described continually in the afternoons they spent alone in the house. Sandra, therefore, although feeling a strong attraction to and curiosity about boys, was very frightened both by the idea of the inevitable clashes with her father, and by the thought that, alone, she might not know how to cope with all the dangers and unknowns that lurked inside boys. The chance was offered her by a female school friend whom she much admired and who, outside the home, was her constant point of reference. This friend, while telling her that there was a boy in the class who like her very much, warmly commended him, several times emphasizing that he was a reliable boy whom one could trust. Sandra felt reassured, as if she were being "entrusted to good hands" by a dependable authority, and this made her want to brave any paternal reactions without delay. This romance, "remote-controlled" at the start, went on for some months. At first, having someone look after her reassured her about her fear of having rows with her father, and made her feel calm and independent from her family. Soon afterward, however, it slowly dawned on her that his solicitous manner was due to a jealousy that was leading him to control any attitudes she had toward her peers. She started "to feel suffocated" when she was at school, and after various qualms and hesitations, abruptly put a stop to this relationship.

With university life first, and later with work, Sandra was able to free herself, partly at least, from family control. She had had a number of relationships with boys and had hence been able to gain experience for herself of the hidden snares of the male world. Her first experience had taught her that one must always seek to gain control of the situation in order not be subject to others, as had happened in her family and with her first boyfriend. So it was always she who made and broke relationships, agilely extricating herself from numerous brief liaisons which she gave no importance to, going from one to the next with apparent nonchalance and self-confidence. The two rela-tionships which, because of the length of time they lasted and the involvement felt, seemed to her to be meaningful were, firstly, from the age of 21 to 23, and secondly, with her present husband, begun at the age of 25. Reconstructing the aspects that these two relationships had in common, and which differentiated them from nonmeaningful ones, her criteria of meaningfulness appeared to be fairly clear: first of all, the partner had to be a strong man, reassuring and authoritative; secondly, although leaning on him unreservedly for support, she nevertheless had to feel that it was she who had control of the relationship. It was exactly this "struggle for control" which seemed at first glance to directly coincide with the level of passion and emotional activation felt in the relationship.

At 21, Sandra was a brilliant woman who had put all the fears and uncertainties of the time of her first experience behind her and who seemed perfectly gratified by her success with the men who seemed to be constantly "at her feet." She, on the one hand, by playing the seductress, kept them "in her orbit" without conceding much, and, on the other, treated them with a haughty air, bored by the fact that she never met a man who could "hold his ground" against her. He, 2 or 3 years older than she, was someone Sandra felt very attracted to and curious about, given that, unlike the others, he seemed immune to her charms. Sandra did everything she could to be at the social events he attended, using her entire seductive repertoire. He, however, feigned such indifference that she perceived it as provocation and hence as a signal of interest. This situation of skirmishing at a distance reached its height when he, coming out into the open, asked her out. Sandra accepted with her usual haughty air, but he did not show up. What should then have been a "settling of accounts" when she, absolutely furious but apparently impassive, went to his house to demand an explanation, instead became an awesome sexual encounter which was the start of their affair. The trend of this relationship, always somewhat tormented, passed through various phases in the course of 2 years before concluding. The first few months seemed to be a continuation of the initial skirmish. Sandra held her ground against his insolence and sarcasm, maintaining situations with other men and giving the general impression that she could leave him for another any time. She was, however, fascinated by his strong, indomitable temperament, so that, despite his apparent unreliability, with no one else did she feel so secure as she did with him. After 5 or 6 months he suddenly changed, and, becoming more and more solicitous and assiduous, asked her for more of her time and involvement. For Sandra, this was equivalent to a sign of victory which left her overjoyed for a couple of months. However, as it gradually began to become clear that his involvement was real, she got a tremendous fright when she suddenly realized that if this affair were to take a "serious" turn, she would no longer be able to do without the security that he transmitted to her. There then began a long phase in which Sandra, precariously poised between the fear of not being able to do without him and that of being alone, started to impose increasing control over her emotions (avoiding intercourse, not reaching orgasm, etc.) and eluded his control (not answering the phone, not showing up for dates, etc.), giving rise to an interminable series of quarrels, arguments, clarifications, and so on. The situation reached its height when he, becoming more and more exasperated, started losing all control in their quarrels, getting drunk and speaking disjointedly. Sandra was horrified to discover that this indomitable man was really a weakling who could not have offered support or protection to anyone. This made her feel progressively stronger, so that during yet another quarrel, she managed to end the situation once and for all. Returning home, however, she felt she had suddenly lost all points of reference. She experienced a moment of bewilderment which turned into a sense of panic so acute that the only way out seemed to be to have herself taken to the emergency department of the nearest hospital. Once she had recovered a degree of control she telephoned her trusted girl friend (the one who had commended her first boyfriend), and as soon as she had accompanied her home, the episode seemed to be closed.

At the age of 25, the "butterfly" period of youth appeared to be by now in second place, and Sandra had started to work with a sense of commitment and responsibility, leading a much more regular life. The previous experience had put her on guard against what she called "contorted people," referring to this last boyfriend, and she hoped for a more tranquil relationship which, as well as guaranteeing the support she felt necessary, would also leave her time and energy to invest in her career.

Her husband was 7 or 8 years older than she, and they had met by chance at work. She was very attracted to him, both because of his strong, decisive ways and because of the imperturbable calm he showed in all things. Although living with another woman, he started a rapid courtship, and Sandra, feeling that his already existing relationship guaranteed that things could not get too serious, wound up by accepting what seemed to her just a brief flirtation. After a few months, however, he brusquely ended his cohabitation and became increasingly solicitous. Sandra once again found herself in a precarious balance between the fear of not being able to let go of him and that of being alone, even though the situation now seemed quite different. The readiness with which her husband had allowed Sandra to control every aspect of his life and the calm he showed at all her extravagances seemed to give her all the necessary guarantees that this would be the right marriage for her. But the more he pressed her for an answer, the more she was unable to decide; this indecision might have gone on for some time had she not become pregnant. It was far simpler to make such an important decision once it became a necessity. Once married, although there were moments of tension because of Sandra's insistence over her independence, which her husband let pass with his usual calm, the menage was fairly tranquil until the emergence of her first panic attack; from that moment on, the structure of the relationship rather abruptly changed, as Sandra could not be alone and required the continual presence of her husband.

Passing the sequence of critical scenes several times "through the moviola" and making use of the ability, which Sandra had by now developed, to reconstruct her subjective experiences by shifting alternately between subjective and objective points of view, it was possible to point out to her the invariant aspects underlying the organization of her affective style.

The connecting thread running through this organization appeared to be centered on a sense of attachment appraised as a need for protection and experienced in antithetical correlation with an equally strong need for freedom and independence. Thus, from the moment of her first love, the sense of feeling protected by a reference figure appeared to be the necessary condition for beginning a relationship. However, as soon as this sense of protection went beyond a certain limit of emotional activation corresponding to the pressure of the partner to intensify the relationship (the "jealousy" of her first boyfriend), the feeling of being limited in her physical and emotional world immediately became the trigger which brought about the breakup of the situation. The commitment to control which emerged from the first experience thus seemed to give her the possibility of better modulating and attenuating the current levels of involvement, correspondingly dampening the fears of constriction and loss of independence. And indeed, as becomes clearer from her relationship at the age of 21, the only cue available for appraising such a complex way of experiencing affectivity was fear, which indiscriminately marked both the beginning of the involvement (fear of losing independence) and the beginning of a disengagement (fear of being alone). In this sense it seemed clear that a competitive interaction, like that which she had at 21, was transformed for her into a setting which "from without" allowed her more control over her involvement, at the same time permitting her to increase at will the level of emotional activation without running the risk of being "dropped." On the other hand, the tormented conclusion of the affair she had begun at 21 made clear, in her eyes, that a competitive setting, on its own, was no longer able to guarantee "a relationship without ties," so that only the "external control" guaranteed by the fact that the partner had another tie seemed to attenuate Sandra's competitiveness, without, however, quenching it entirely (e.g., quarrels about independence, difficulty of making a decision about marriage proportional to his insistence). This need for outside control was also evident in the possibility, provided by the "unexpected" pregnancy, of finally being able to decide to tie herself to someone.

Finally, feelings linked to a disengagement or to an increased emotional detachment seemed to become partly recognizable due to a concomitant change of image of the partner from "strong" to "weak" (which is what happened in her relationship at the age of 21 and in that with her husband, as we have seen above). The emotions linked to a greater involvement in a situation instead seemed to be less recognizable and could be experienced only as an uncontrollable fear of losing control over herself, the most evident situation being that with her husband, in which she had reacted to his detachment (discovery of betrayal) by obliging him to stay in continual contact with her (and thus putting herself in a situation of greater involvement); however, it was almost impossible for her at the outset of therapy to trace what she felt to the emotional reciprocity going on with her husband.

As we have seen, for Winnie the affective relationship experienced as essential in her present life structure was the relationship with her mother. So in this case one was not dealing so much with analyzing a "sentimental career," which in practice had yet to begin, as with reconstructing the current self-organization of her affective style from the way in which she had structured her relationship with her mother. As the reformulation of the original problem, undertaken in the work done so far, gradually clarified, it became clearer for

Winnie that what should be reconstructed was the way in which she had structured a relationship with her mother which did not allow even the slightest reappraisal of her image.

For Winnie the current trend of the relationship with her mother had started when she was 15, from the beginning of high school. During the 3 years of middle school she felt able to cope with her mother, even to the point of having furious rows with her. By mutual agreement it was therefore decided to begin to analyze her experiencing of her relationship with her mother starting from the middle school period (age 12 on), in order to be able to reconstruct the way in which such experiencing had later changed. The critical events, broken down into corresponding scenes, would be "put through the moviola" several times; they were arranged, roughly speaking, as follows:

Her mother had always presented herself as an exemplary woman in her roles of wife and mother, continually complaining that her husband and daughters did not have the feelings, strength of will, and ability equal to her own. With this continual attitude of pointing out the "negativity" of the other members of the family with respect to her "positivity," her mother several times emphasized that they all weighed heavily on her shoulders, with the result that she had always sacrificed herself for those who did not deserve it. Everyone in the family had always accepted this formulation of things and had put themselves out, in the hope not so much of meeting the mother's expectations (which seemed impossible) as, if nothing else, of not disappointing her too much and thus managing to alleviate the weight of a sacrifice made inevitable by their incompetence.

For Winnie, everything started to change when she was 12, at the beginning of middle school. Not that she cast her mother's sacrificial role into doubt, but she had simply begun all of a sudden to appraise the atmosphere at home as suffocating and felt oppressed. So she began to react to her mother's criticisms, at first with spirited protests which ended up with "tears of guilt" in her room, and then, gradually, with real clashes in which Winnie alternated tears with fury. If one broadened the focus of exploration in order to include other experiential domains, one could clearly see how this changed attitude toward her mother went in parallel with other changes which had come about in the meantime.

Winnie went to middle school late because of years lost due to illness in elementary school, so this change coincided with a true

"change of world" which did not derive simply from the increased complexity of scholastic level and the consequently greater diligence required. In the first place, Winnie spent almost her whole day at school as her mother, to lighten the load of bringing up the family on her own, expected her daughter to do her homework at school. This had put her into closer contact with the world of her peers, which seemed different and fascinating. Secondly, with her literature mistress, whom Winnie esteemed greatly and considered exceptional, she had from the beginning established an affectionate and cordial relationship. This teacher, once lessons were over, stayed behind to talk to Winnie in the garden and showing herself to be always very understanding, stimulated her interests and curiosity, encouraging her to follow them up. While this relationship became more permanent and friendly, Winnie found herself facing totally new experiences; she was not a little amazed to feel herself to be understood instead of criticized in the daily rows that she was having with her mother. So while the family atmosphere continued to be more and more suffocating, school had become the only place in which Winnie felt at ease, to the point where she awaited the arrival of Sunday with anxiety. In this way, her teacher eventually became transformed for Winnie into an absolute model of reference, so that for the whole period of middle school she tried to be like her in all things, even taking on her most banal attitudes and gestures.

When, at 15, at the end of middle school, she changed schools and started high school, the trend of things at home had not changed; on the contrary, the rows with her mother had increased because of the new exigencies of adolescence which Winnie now claimed. The situation came brusquely to a head, however, one afternoon when during one of the usual rows, her mother, absolutely beside herself, threatened to shut her up in a boarding school known for its severity until she was of age. Winnie was terrified both by the seriousness of the threat and by the fact that her mother, usually so composed, had lost control of herself in that way. She immediately felt that in this struggle of hers, which all of a sudden seemed senseless to her, she must have done something irreparable; she felt "defeated" and "nullified," and bursting into tears, implored her mother to forgive her, declaring herself ready to do anything as long as she did so. Shortly afterwards it was finished, and no more mention was made of boarding school. However, from that moment Winnie began more and more often to feel "empty" and incapable of feeling sensations, and, in parallel, her attitude toward her mother changed radically. Winnie no longer reacted to her criticisms, but changed into a girl dedicated to study and to the family, as if being thought of as her mother's right hand had become her only ambition. From then on, save the momentary disagreement over her brief flirtation during the summer when she was 17, the relationship with her mother stayed within these lines.

Passing the individual scenes "through the moviola" several times and relying on the ability that Winnie now had both to differentiate between the sense of self and the behavior of others, and to see herself in the same scene from the inside and from the outside, it was possible to show how it had progressively become unbearable for her to experience any reappraisal of her mother's perceived image.

The point of departure in the scene-analysis procedure was that of reconstructing the role played in the affective domain by an aspect which had seemed notable to Winnie from preceding work, that is, the "externally bound" attitude of mirroring herself in others' behavior to be able to self-refer and recognize her immediate experiencing. In this way it began to become clear to her that such an attitude was inherent in her way of structuring affective relationships.

On the one hand, perceiving the other as an absolute model was the essential criterion for a person to be experienced as significant; on the other, being attuned with and adhering to his or her perceived expectations was the essential way to feel herself involved in an exclusive relationship while at the same time experiencing a definite sense of herself. Focusing particularly on this aspect, going back and forth in the sequence of critical scenes, it became fairly straightforward to emphasize how her sense of self changed radically according to whether the reference model was represented by her mother or by her teacher.

Secondly, it seemed essential that in her "existential horizon" there should always be an absolute model of reference available and that the changes taking place within her (need for more autonomy from her mother and sharing more in the world of her peers) eventually coincided with the passage from one reference model to another. Indeed, if one reconstructed the period in which she was able to stand up to her mother, it soon became evident that this corresponded to the period in which she experienced the privileged relationship with her teacher. Continuing to focus on this period, it became easy to see that her distancing herself from a model did not consist so much of modifying her way of representing it, but rather of trying to substitute it almost mechanically from "outside" with another that at the time seemed to her more valid. In fact, if one reconstructed her subjective experience during the rows of the middle school period, one could see that there was no trace of criticism of her mother's way of doing things which she still considered valid. What was happening in her was simply that she was trying to oppose, as a test of strength, the image, attitudes, and opinions of her teacher against her mother's way of doing things. In this test of strength she slowly felt herself losing from the moment that she changed school and the relationship with her teacher, no longer a daily matter, became progressively redimensioned.

It then became equally clear what had happened on that famous afternoon in which, all of a sudden, she had felt defeated and nullified and which she immediately attributed to some intrinsic incompetence (as her mother had always said). Being no longer able to oppose the image of her teacher to that of her mother she suddenly felt as if she were deprived of any possible identity, and this, more than the threat of boarding school, had frightened her to death. At that point, only an even more unconditional adherence to the model represented by her mother—who, apart from anything else, was the only one available to her—could enable her to glimpse a possible way out of that sense of indefiniteness of self which she appraised as intolerable. All this naturally brought with it a whole range of self-deceptive mechanisms which seemed to guarantee the possibility of recognizing herself in an absolute reference model, but which in actual fact further diminished the possibility of reaching a stable and definite sense of self. On the one hand, the more she exerted herself to exclude feelings and opinions that could interfere with her attunement to her mother's expectations, the more intense and pervasive became the sense of emptiness and the fear of not feeling any emotions. On the other hand, every time (as in the period of her summer flirtation) the experiencing of a change in the mother's image circumvented her deceptive self-referring, its emerging into consciousness could only be appraised as an absolutely unbearable calling into question of herself.

It should finally be pointed out that while the reconstruction of her affective style proceeded, passing the sequence of critical scenes "through the moviola," there was carried on, in parallel, a reframing of these same scenes in which the image of her mother as a person was reconstructed, using Winnie's new ability to differentiate her mother's behavior from her own sense of self. This reframing was marked by a consistent reappraisal of the image of the mother whose "being a victim of others' inadequacy" seemed more and more to Winnie to be a mask through which the mother managed to manipulate all the members of the family without ever coming out into the open with her need for control and power in relationships.

The affect-laden events that characterized Gregory's affective history—reconstructed according to the usual points in order—gave rise to the following picture:

Following a difficult puberty studded with various dilemmas as to the rightness or otherwise of sexual impulses (erotic fantasies, masturbation, etc.), Gregory went through adolescence fairly secluded from his peers, as only being with the family seemed to lift him out of the various doubts pervading him. His sentimental debut took place at the age of 19–20 and coincided with the first time Gregory spent a summer holiday at camp with some people of his own age. They got to know the other boys and girls from neighboring tents and Gregory found himself more and more frequently in the company of two very active and enterprising sisters who involved him in nearly all their enterprises. At first, Gregory accepted their invitations somewhat timidly and awkwardly so as not to disappoint them, then he gradually began to feel at ease because of their vivacity and spontaneity, so that he realized, and was disoriented by it, that he felt something for them which was perhaps more than just simple liking. In a state of growing tension, Gregory felt, for a moment, that he was absolutely unable to control his sexual impulses, feeling himself pervaded by the usual tormenting doubts about himself (wicked/nonwicked, etc.). He seemed to recover a margin of control over this intolerable sense of perhaps being a despicable person, as he gradually persuaded himself that the only way to be "serious" and "perfect" was to choose which of the two sisters seemed the "right" one in terms of strength of feeling and human values. The result was that the more he weighed the pros and cons, the more uncertain he felt, and if he tried to call on the sisters for help, explaining his doubts, he was overwhelmed by a wave of hilarity and joking that left him even more diffident and anxious. The situation came to a head one morning as he was explaining his usual doubts to one of the sisters, seeking reassurance and con-firmation; at first she pretended to be listening, and then, jumping over to him, kissed him passionately and then ran away laughing herself helpless. Gregory felt betrayed and cheated, and became even colder and more detached. Another reason for this behavior was that the sudden kiss had produced unforeseen sensations in him which once again evoked doubts about himself. Fortunately, his holiday soon finished and Gregory, returning to his usual, reassuring daily life, soon classified the experience as an anomaly attributable to the promiscuity inherent in such situations—which from now on he would assiduously avoid.

After this experience, Gregory threw himself into his studies, and his relationship with girls consisted of brief flirtations which started out full of ideals and noble values and which immediately disappointed him because of their sensual charge, leaving him still more wary and diffident. Reviewing his sentimental career as a whole, two meaningful relationships could be identified: the first from 21 to 22, and the second with his wife, begun at 23. The criteria for meaningfulness recognizable in both situations were that the partner should be much more exuberant and spontaneous in her emotivity than him, and moreover that such emotivity, combined with other gifts, should be capable of arousing in him total commitment, devoid of all imperfection or uncertainty.

In the first relationship, at age 21–22, he had met the girl at university and had immediately been attracted by her vitality and ease of manner, and so he gradually became more assiduous, courting her in a very veiled and embarrassed way. This would probably have followed the course of his flirtations, which he began enthusiastically and quickly grew cold, had she not presented him with a *fait accompli* by saying in front of everyone that they were dating. Gregory felt at that moment quite unable to react given that, on the one hand, he appraised it as an exalting confirmation of her interest, but, on the other hand, he also felt it as a weight that had fallen on him and which he would have to bear. For the moment, the exalting aspect seemed to hold sway and he decided that this was a "joyous weight" and accepted being launched into a relationship. Slowly, however, the weight, though joyous, began to weigh heavier, so that he started to progressively detach himself, reflecting and ruminating over the best way to end the situation. All his ruminating came to a halt, however, when faced with the fact that breaking off the relationship would mean making her suffer, as she always seemed so enthusiastic and involved. In this way, surrounded by doubts and long silences when they were together, the relationship dragged on for nearly a year, until she, exasperated, decided to break off what by now seemed

to her an irretrievable situation. Gregory was not too upset by her
departure, nor by what she had said when she broke up with him;
indeed, many times he had imagined this as a possible way things
might go, and this all seemed to him perfectly understandable. He
therefore promised himself once more to be cautious and prudent in
his search for the right situation.

The occasion when he met his wife, at university once again,
had been preceded by a very brief summer flirtation with an English
girl who for a moment had seemed to him to correspond completely to
his ideal woman; the disappointment had then so embittered him that
he dismissed the importance of everything he had believed until that
moment, and had shelved the matter.

Gregory had been attracted by her emotional temperament, at
once lively and reassuring, and by the uncommon intelligence he had
glimpsed in his wife; thus, little by little it became clear that this could
finally be the relationship that he had been looking for, so much so
that, contrary to his usual habits, it was he who took the initiative to
start this relationship.

However, as the relationship was taking a more involving turn,
largely because of his wife's enthusiasm and enterprise, Gregory began
to have pervasive and tormenting doubts as to whether the right
woman was in fact his wife or the English girl, who had suddenly
reappeared from memory. Months of uncertainty followed, during
which he continually ruminated on the comparison between the two
while thrown into doubt about setting out, despite himself, on a path
which might in the end prove to be the wrong one. His wife's
reassurances grew more attentive and solicitous, and her family
showed themselves to be ready to welcome him among them, so these
doubts, at a certain point, began to wane. It therefore seemed the
obvious thing to everybody when during the engagement party, his
father-in-law, who was of the same profession that Gregory was soon
to start, proposed that he join his firm as soon as he graduated. The
tranquility thus achieved lasted only briefly. As we saw in the first part
of this chapter, as the date of the wedding drew near, Gregory began
to have innumerable doubts about the ceremony, the dates, and so on,
which, following his wife's ultimatum, led to the frightening insight of
possibly being the unwitting victim of someone else's game of opportunity.

Passing the individual scenes "through the moviola" and relying
on the ability, which Gregory now possessed, to differentiate between

experiencing and explaining, as well as that of being able to reconstruct the multifaceted aspects of ongoing feelings while observing himself from within and from without, it was possible to reconstruct the invariants underlying his way of structuring affective relationships.

His difficulty in recognizing complex emotions became clear to him, especially unfolding ones (e.g., a progressive engagement or an emerging disengagement). This is what happened, although with different intensity, in his first experience and in his relationship with his wife; in the second relationship, where the involvement felt by him was somewhat reduced, the doubts and fears had concerned, through his anticipatory ruminations, the management and control of the emotions which separation might have evoked.

Focusing on individual scenes, it became clear that this difficulty depended on the assumption that emotions behaved with the same unequivocality and coherence as thoughts; in fact the moment he appraised the slightest contrasting aspect in his feelings, this, with the coherence of his "all-or-nothing" logic, was immediately experienced as something calling both himself and the relationship into question. Thus, even the smallest displeasure he felt immediately meant that the partner was not the right one, and that he had yet again made a mistake. If, therefore, he found himself in some flirtation with no commitment, he let it drop and was left feeling disappointed; in an already established relationship, however, the displeasure, if not immediately "erased" and deprived of all validity, gave rise to doubts and uncertainties which protracted into continual ruminating.

Finally, it was equally evident that this difficulty in self-referring feelings and emotions was linked to the continual worry of maintaining an image of himself which was acceptable in terms of his extremely rigid ethical and moral principles. Focusing on individual scenes, the continuity of these self-deceptive mechanisms became, even in his eyes, ever clearer: the causal external attribution with which he explained the trend of his flirtations (e.g., promiscuity); or the breakup of his relationships (e.g., his second relationship) which allowed him to shelve everything without having to revise his image of himself; or, finally, the avoidance of direct self-referral of "negative" feelings, such as resentment or hostility toward his wife, with the result (as seen in the first part of the chapter) of excessively multiplying his ruminations and doubts about himself.

It is clear that in a work of reconstruction of this nature more effective results in triggering a change in the client's current viewpoint on him- or herself are related to the therapist's knowledge of the dynamics of various organizations of personal meaning (P.M.Orgs.).

On the one hand, knowing that any P.M.Org., when experiencing an affective imbalance, is characterized by specific distressing feelings as well as by equally specific self-deceiving patterns orients the therapist in understanding the difficulties emerging from deepening self-observation and in shifting the focus toward those patterns of coherence not accessible to the client.

On the other hand, knowing how any P.M.Org. unfolds through lifespan development helps the therapist formulate hypotheses both about the nature of the imbalance that has occurred and about its effects on the corresponding existential period, and consequently to elaborate strategies more effective in reordering disruptive feelings. Hence, there is undoubtedly a different intensity and quality to disturbing emotions produced by the unbalancing of a relationship already established in one's life structure (Richard and Sandra) with respect to one which still seems to be in the initial stages (Gregory). All this is even more apparent in Winnie's case, where the elaboration of a strategy required from the therapist the knowledge of the difficulty of emotional distancing from parents usually exhibited during adolescence by eating-disorders-prone subjects; that is, knowing how an unbalancing in the relationship with the mother could be matched by a lack of emotional detachment and sense of autonomy from that figure, it becomes possible to plan the reconstruction of the relationship with the mother in such a way as to facilitate the relativization of her figure which turned out to still be at the beginning stage.

Finally, going back and forth through critical events with the usual scene-analysis procedure during the whole reconstruction of an affective style (varying between a minimum of 3 to a maximum of 7 months) brings about a gradual reordering of immediate experiences paralleled by a reframing of these same events. This, in turn, triggers off a further appreciable change in the client's viewpoint on him- or herself (change in the "Me" appraisal of the "I").

At this stage it consists of a shifting from experiencing the repetitiveness of affective events as "given as such" to appraising it as a self-organized procedure aimed at maintaining one's perceived sense of self through the ongoing production of recurrent feelings and emotional tonalities consistent with the experiencing of one's continuity and uniqueness. This change in the "Me" appraisal of the "I" is matched by the emergence of a second level of restructuring of the range of perceivable emotions: on the one hand, the client can recognize and appreciate how different emotional states combine and recombine themselves when going through an affectional bond, just as the perception of a significant other comes to regulate his or her self-perception; on the other hand, he or she is now able to experience how these recombinations and perceptions of significant others unfold through a personal meaning coherence whose traces are now recognizable from early developmental periods on.

As well as being accompanied by a practically total disappearance of the original disturbances, a change in the viewpoint of oneself of this kind brings the emergence of new levels of abstract self-referring in ordering past and present experiences, and a different attitude toward reality with the discovery of new experiential domains. It may thus be understandable that more than 50% of clients prefer to stop at this point of the treatment, maintaining a relationship with the therapist through check-up sessions which gradually decrease in frequency (e.g., first once a month, then every 2 or 3, then every 5 or 6, and so on) and cease altogether, generally speaking, in the space of 2 or 3 years. It is clear that the therapist should have no qualms about the client stopping at this point in the work; indeed, there does not exist an unequivocal way in which things should unfold (including the therapy being carried out) and the client remains, in the final analysis, the only one who can decide what is the best way for him or her to proceed along his or her life trajectory.

8

Undertaking the Developmental Analysis

INTRODUCTORY REMARKS

The third phase lasts between a minimum of 3 to a maximum of 6 months, and thus takes place in the second year of therapy. This phase begins when clients are interested in continuing personal exploration despite the disappearance of the disturbances that were troubling them. Generally it is only necessary to clarify the work of self-observation which they are preparing to undertake. At this point, it is clear to clients that their goal is to reconstruct the way in which their developmental pathway led them to structure that personal meaning which became so clear in their eyes during the completion of the second phase.

The first step consists of reconstructing the client's developmental history in order to identify the significant events to be broken down into their corresponding scenes which will subsequently be passed "through the moviola" repeatedly. This is certainly not a simple matter for the therapist, and not only because memories of the past, despite their importance, are often vague, imprecise, and superimposed on one another. The main difficulty is that the client usually endorses a version of his or her past history which has been "tidying itself up" over the years with *ad hoc* explanations that appear to be in keeping with a specific image of oneself, although it has been undergoing modification during the second phase of therapy.

Despite the different characteristics depending on the type of meaning organization, what one finds, almost invariably, is that the affect-laden attachment memories, deceptively appraised and self-referred, are characterized by explanations which are discrepant with the experiencing that such memories trigger off. Given that the explanations appear to be more consistent with their perceived coherence, clients usually assume that "the facts" are identified with the explanations rather than with their experiencing. Making continual reference to the experiencing/explaining differentiation during the reconstruction allows the therapist to recognize the significant discrepant scenes to be reordered and at the same time to make what the client had taken for granted seem different. Therefore, rather than by the insistence with which certain topics are presented or the motives adduced ("explaining"), the events to be considered significant should instead be identified by the type of emotional resonance they give rise to ("experiencing") and by the way in which the client manages to recognize and self-refer it. In this way, the memories which appear to be significant are those which, regardless of the "obviousness" or "banality" of their content, arouse "discrepant" sensations and emotions, that is, those for which the client cannot give what he or she feels is an exhaustive explanation. Once again, therefore, it is knowledge of the stages of development characterizing the self-organization of personal meaning dimensions, added to the knowledge of the specific deceptive ways with which the client self-refers immediate experiencing, that guides the therapist in identifying the significant events on which to focus.

Therefore, starting from the very earliest memories of life that it is possible to recall, one proceeds with a thorough gathering of affect-laden events, analyzing in succession the trend of the main maturational stages, that is, *infancy and preschool years* (from 0 to 6); *childhood* (from around 7 to 12–13); *adolescence and youth* (from 13 to 20–21) (see Appendix).

The interdependence between attachment and selfhood processes (and the way in which this interdependence regulates the interplay between emotional differentiation and cognitive growth) is the developmental thread which provides the self-observational focus in going back and forth in the sequence of affect-laden scenes. Thus, for each scene, one puts into focus both the sequence of interactions contained therein in order to reconstruct the attachment patterns in progress, and the subjective experience of the child in order to reconstruct the sense of self and of the world appraised at that moment.

The scene-analysis procedure essentially remains the same as in the preceding phases, with the only difference that, making use of the client's advanced skills in the self-observational method, the reconstruction of a significant experience at a certain age may be carried out while further broadening the continuous shifting between subjective and objective viewpoints. Indeed, once the subjective viewpoint with which an event was experienced has been reconstructed, it can be matched against two different objective viewpoints:

1. How one would see him- or herself from without with the "eyes" of that same age (thus being able to reconstruct with greater thoroughness the sensations felt and the consequent discoveries which were at the time held to have been made).
2. How one sees now from without while focusing on that age, reconstructing with "eyes of the present" (i.e., from the changed viewpoint which has emerged in the preceding phase) the discoveries which, from those sensations, *one now thinks one made then.*

As the focus of the exploration gradually deepens, the self-observation viewpoints increase, and it is precisely this continuous and alternating shifting between viewpoints throughout the developmental analysis that allows the client's flexibility to increase to the point where it triggers further changes in his or her current viewpoint on him- or herself.

In describing the developmental analysis of our clients, we shall describe only the salient moments of the reconstruction under way, that is, those in which the client experienced an intense emotional activation in focusing on certain events and those in which there came about a reframing of memories which were particularly critical in the development of personal meaning. It is as well to bear in mind, however, that the therapeutic efficacy of any developmental analysis depends not only on the reframing of critical memories (undoubtedly essential), but also on the amount of time spent on the methodical and repetitive going back and forth in order to increase the client's flexibility.

CASE ILLUSTRATIONS

Richard was able to trace that sense of sadness which had always accompanied him to his earliest memories of life, going back to 2 or 3 years of age. He attributed his sadness to the fact this his parents had had him at a fairly late age, when they had already resigned themselves to not having children and to leading an existence without pretensions or excitement, in the company of a much older housekeeper who looked after them. His first images of life were of "grey surroundings" and "gloomy atmospheres" in which there moved old people whom he appraised as "lifeless" and entirely detached from his child's world. In these first years, it was not possible to trace any image of his interacting with other people, whether playing games with other children or with adults. His most tranquil moments were those spent alone in the garden, whereas in contact with his parents he was always perturbed by their economic vicissitudes, which they talked about continually. The clearest memory of this time was when he was 4, and concerned his father, who, leaning toward him and with a worried look on his face, said, "How are we going to be able to give you a future with the situation we're in?" This was a memory that still perturbed him deeply, so much so that every time he talked about it, his voice was broken by tears. It was the first time that it had become clear to him that his birth had turned out to be an unbearable burden for his parents, who otherwise would have been able to lead a peaceful life undisturbed by life's troubles.

Focusing on all the scenes with his mother or with his father, one was struck by the total lack of any moment whatever of emotional contact or effusion with his parents. Richard attributed this to his parents being taken up by "far more important things than slobbering over their son." Indeed, with his birth they had had to intensify their work which proceeded in the midst of difficulties and uncertainties, and, in addition, he had been, from the start, a "sickly" child, and as such, a continual source of worry which eventually and inevitably took the place of carefree moments of affection which might otherwise have been possible.

Because of his delicate health, he was forced to forgo nursery school and put off the long-awaited moment of meeting his peers until the beginning of school. However, just before the beginning of primary school, the family doctor found that he had a "weak heart" and dissuaded his parents from sending him to school. Consequently, during the primary school years, Richard stayed at home to study, aided by an elderly retired teacher who came wearily to him every day with the sole obvious aim of adding to a somewhat meager pension. This additional unforeseen expense naturally worsened the already precarious family budget, and Richard appraised this as his weighing even further on his old and tired parents who surely deserved quite a different son. He appraised this particularly with his father, a figure who aroused tenderness and respect at the same time as being seen as always "unreachable" and taken up with worries of which he was largely the cause. It was above all for his father (whom he referred to affectionately as "my Old Man") that he had decided to make as much effort as possible in his studies in order to be able in that way to repay him, at least in part, for all the troubles he had unwittingly brought into the home. Richard asserted that he did not much feel the effects of those years of isolation and lack of amusement because of this total commitment to his studies, which gave him a sense of being one of the family. When at the age of 11 he took the exams for entry to middle school, he came out top, and received a cash prize which he proudly presented to his father with the sense of finally having "earned" his place in the family.

However, toward the age of 12, his "weakness of the heart" seemed to have been overcome, and his parents, stressing that this was yet another sacrifice, decided to send him to a fairly renowned board-ing school where he would be able to obviate the inevitable lacunae of private study. Although he made an effort not to give anything away, Richard appraised the imminent separation from his parents with a deep sense of desperation and with the pervasive anxiety that he would perhaps not see them again. At the moment of getting on the train, his mother in saying goodbye embraced and kissed him for the first time; the moment he realized that this had never happened before, Richard had the confirmation that this was a matter of defini-tive, irreversible separation, and burst into uncontrollable tears, de-spite his father's repeatedly urging him to "be a man."

Initially, installing himself in his new surroundings was ex-tremely difficult. He arrived in college with the reputation of being "clever" but "different" and "sickly," which did not put him in a good light with his fellows; and also the impact with this world, which in comparison to home seemed so complex, had been so sudden that Richard, unequipped with even the most elementary norms of social behavior, felt clumsy and awkward and mostly kept to himself. So, as he realized with dismay that he would have to go it alone anyway, he involved himself more and more in his studies and immersed himself in literature, which allowed him to "live parallel lives in books."

Although remaining at the top scholastically, he gradually man-aged to make himself appreciated and accepted by his peers, eventually becoming an indisputable leader. This period from age 13 to 15 corresponded to a period of well-being that Richard had never felt before, and of discoveries he had never imagined. From contact with his peers he had discovered he had qualities that others appreciated and that it was therefore possible for him to feel differently about himself from how he felt at home. From the occasional contact with the families of his peers who came to visit (and at whom he gazed through astonished eyes) he had discovered, with even more wonder, a whole way of being and of seeing the world which was different from that experienced at home.

From age 15 to 17, Richard, continuing in his role as leader, suddenly started to do less well at school, something he could not explain even as an adult except by attributing it to a "reawakening of the senses" which he began to feel overwhelmingly during that period. When his father, on his rare visits, treated him coldly as if he were a "degenerate," Richard felt a mixture of humiliation, remorse, and rage which threw him into the blackest despair for weeks afterwards.

The situation came to a head when he was nearly 18 and his father withdrew him from his boarding school in order to send him to another one which was much stricter and more rigorous. Richard at first felt despair at the news, and then suddenly had an attack of fury he had never imagined possible. In the grip of uncontrollable turmoil he refused to go to college or even to continue with school and shut himself up in his room, immersing himself as much as possible in the literature that had become his "real life."

There followed a year of tension and despair. From that moment, his father did not speak to him again and spoke of him in the past as if he were dead, even though he silently consented to the fact that "unknown to him," the mother sent food and a little money to his room. Richard could not understand how his father could behave as if he did not exist and now felt a sense of "cosmic" solitude, when as a child he had felt merely a burden. He also felt that all his attempts to be different had been useless folly, and that the only thing that might have mattered, "making an effort for the Old Man's sake," had turned out to be a colossal failure for which he alone, as usual, was responsible. So, at the age of 19 or 20, when after his disappointing first love experience it seemed that nothing justified his continuing presence there, he decided to play to the full his role as degenerate son and abandoned his family amidst general opposition. As now became clear, this role had allowed him for years to daydream about the day when as a famous director he would return home welcomed with affection, recognition, and his father's apologies. The fact that both his parents died when he was still a long way from establishing himself as a director confirmed for him that he had been a disgrace for them, and that he might also be a disgrace for all those who loved him.

Repeatedly passing "through the moviola" the ensemble of affect-laden scenes, it was a fairly straightforward matter to reconstruct the gradual self-organization of Richard's depressive meaning, while at the same time reordering his appraisal of the past.

For Richard it was clear that, from the first stages of life, solitude and the sense of affective loss (i.e., not deserving the affection and attention of his parents because of having "ruined" their life) represented the connecting thread along which his entire history had unfolded. What was less clear was how the attachment dynamics influenced all this and the role played by his parents. As is entirely characteristic in the process of encoding and assembling memories by helpless children (see Chapter 3), Richard had the tendency to minimize the experience of distressing affect (the almost total isolation of childhood was not considered particularly stressing) as well as the tendency to dismiss the importance of the relationship with his parents as a source of comfort or support ("they had more important things to think about"). Moreover, it was just this tendency to reduce or exclude the perceived level of affect which made it possible for certain memories to be accompanied by feelings which, not meeting with adequate appraisal and self-referring, still had a perturbing effect.

The memory belonging to the age of 4, which still made him cry whenever he talked about it, was particularly indicative in this sense, and passing it "through the moviola" several times was for Richard an intense emotional experience accompanied by various discoveries about himself and his parents. If while working with the experiencing/ explaining differentiation, at which Richard was by now proficient, one "took seriously" the sense of helplessness, that is, that as immediate experience this was *the fact* to be explained, the perspective with which to put the scene into focus became: What attitude of the father had made it possible that helplessness should become for him the most suitable "reading"? Shifting continuously in seeing from within and without (from both objective viewpoints) both himself and his father, it became clear that what had struck him most about his father's attitude was his "making him a participant in the problems of the household, as if he were an adult" which he had appraised as a crushing responsibility; the "weight," therefore, was that of not being able to be a child, experienced as the impossibility of having (i.e., loss) the protection, affection, and attention due to a child. Moreover, if the focus was broadened, running up and down the whole sequence of critical images of childhood, one saw how this theme of "not deserving the affection due to children," confirmed moment by moment by the total lack of affection on the part of his parents, was being articulated; on the one hand, protecting his parents from the "disgrace" which he represented allowed him, at the time, to recover at least in part some reciprocal affection, while leaving open the possibility that "making a big effort for his folks" would one day fully recover this affection (inversion of the parent–child relationship). On the other hand, he was able to look after himself efficiently in situations which would be difficult for any other child, such as that of pursuing his studies alone during his childhood and still managing to come out on top (self-caring and compulsive self-reliance). Moreover, as these different aspects began to tie up, it became clearer for Richard that his parents' behavior—attribution of heavy responsibility coupled with the lack of emotional support needed to deal with it—rather than depending on their advanced age, instead corresponded to a rigid strategy of upbringing which allowed them to have complete control over him with the minimum of emotional investment (so-called "parental affectionless control"). In order for a strategy of this nature to maintain its efficacy over the years with the minimum of effort, it was necessary that the moment any responsibility had been fulfilled, another was immediately presented which required even more effort and devotion. When Richard thought he had managed to "earn a place in the home" with the brilliant exam results for admission to middle school, he suddenly found himself alone on a train to boarding school, an event which seemed more than he could handle. In this way, the experience of never having been able to attain a secure emotional attachment had slowly become the central aspect of his "world," and loneliness, anger, a sense of unlovableness, and so on, the specific ways of recognizing and self-referring his "being-in-it." Thus, the experiencing of helplessness, anger, etc., besides providing the continuity of his patterns of self-perception, was also a generative way of structuring new experiential domains, such as, for example, studying, the passion for literature, the construction of a repertoire of social skills, and so on.

If one shifted the focus onto his "fall" in school results between the ages of 15 and 17, it became clear that, first, his discoveries about himself had begun to distinguish those themes and interests which would subsequently be developed, first in his life as a journalist and then as a director, and second, the discovery that another world from that of home was possible, which, as well as arousing resentment and anger toward his father, had brought him to feel more and more that devotion or commitment as such were useless effort. It was clear to him during those years that the exaggerated effort should have been aimed at feeling differently from how he felt at home, and even if working as a director seemed an unattainable goal, managing to try and go it alone seemed far more praiseworthy and more able to reconcile him with the world at large. It seemed to him that the sense of despair and humiliation he felt in the face of the coldness of his father was the price to pay to his Old Man in order to deserve the way he had chosen to follow, and that the Old Man would in the end have understood and appreciated his son's interests.

Faced with the sudden decision to change boarding schools, he felt he had lost everything, the present world he believed he had conquered and the old world he believed he belonged to, and that he had become a stranger to his father. As his anger gradually diminished, the despair became so intense as to make him feel he could only mitigate it by suicide or a complete withdrawal from the world.

If one ran the subsequent period "through the moviola," it became evident to him, first, that his father's attitude, pretending he did not know how to support him, was none other than a power maneuver to bring him back under control; second, it seemed clear to him that he had appraised this separation as a real abandonment, similar to what he felt with his wife, and in the same way, excessively intensifying the sense of his negativity, he had tried to maintain in some way an emotional tie to his "Old Man." The role of the "degenerate" son, in fact, making him feel he was the only person responsible for what had happened, permitted him to maintain the image of his father intact, thus preserving emotional reciprocity with him, and at the same time being able to fight with all his strength to restore a full relationship with him, as is demonstrated in exemplary fashion by his fantasy of "the prodigal son."

It was precisely at this point that Richard realized how feeling himself to be the only one responsible for the separation which had for so many years existed between himself and his father had prevented him from realizing that, although his father had always had news of him and knew where he was living, *not once* did he seek him out in all those years, not even taking the trouble to utilize all those various circumstantial reasons which would not have altered his (the father's) role of the "offended party." The dismay he felt at never having noticed something so blindingly obvious diminished gradually as Richard realized that, in order to maintain his image of his father, he could not allow himself to see the obvious. It became clear to him that his father had always felt him to be an extraneous intrusion, and that only that viewpoint could explain the absence of even the most elemental paternal feelings, which usually arise spontaneously.

This sudden realization and the consequent change in perspective of his father corresponded to a fairly intense emotional situation, so much so that at the end of the session, Richard could not hold back his tears, tears which had begun submissively with the usual sense of irreparable loss (in this case, of having wasted his life for a person who had never felt him to be his son) and which gradually became a sense of being deeply moved and exalted in feeling himself released from that sense of solitude and personal ruin which had as its base the certainty that he had always made the only people who loved him suffer.

Sandra had always maintained that her fear of being alone or of losing control had "fallen from the sky" onto her when she was already grown up. This had always made her think, in agreement with the general opinion at home, that these fears therefore depended on some sort of "constitutional fragility" which had gradually emerged toward puberty and adolescence. In fact she had led a carefree and "idyllic" childhood, in touch with nature, as her parents were farmers who worked in a small valley in the South where there was no electricity and where life had remained in an almost natural state.

Her first images of life evoked a sense of serenity and tranquility and mostly concerned the farm on which they lived (and which was shared with her paternal grandparents by whom she had been much indulged) and the attentions and solicitations of her mother, her main emotional figure of reference, given that her father was always out in the fields.

Indeed, one memory, dated at 3 or 4 years of age, that seemed to stand out from the others concerned her mother. It was a summer afternoon and she was out in the fields with her mother on one of those occasions (threshing, or whatever) in which all the women of the village came out to help the men. In the important scene, Sandra was near her mother who, in order not to bore her, was making her little dolls out of earth which broke as soon as she, Sandra, took them in her hands, at which her mother, with the patience of a saint, immediately began to make her another one, although reproached by her father, who would have preferred that she spend more time on her work. Sandra gradually felt the sense of protection and affection that surrounded her diminish, giving way to a rising tide of irritation and anger that frightened her enormously, so that she burst into tears, clinging to her mother's skirts. She seemed somewhat perturbed in reporting this memory, and explained the irritation and anger with the fact that her mother did not know how to make earth dolls that did not immediately break. Clinging to her mother's skirts in tears she attributed to the fright she got in feeling herself to be so ungrateful in the face of such affection.

When she was 5 it was decided to send her to nursery school in a village a few miles away and to which her grandfather had offered to take her every day. The first day, Sandra felt herself a little out of place and frightened, and never left her teacher's side. Although she had anxiously awaited the moment, on returning she made no mention of this to her grandfather, as he would have reported it to her father whose brusque ways she feared. She held it all in until they got home and ran straight to her mother saying that she did not want to go to nursery school anymore. Her mother reassured her and then confronted her husband and father-in-law and got them to agree that her daughter should stop going to nursery school.

This episode marked for Sandra the beginning of a "complicity" with her mother which was to last until the latter's death and which always gave her the sense of being a privileged child, more loved and understood than others. She, for her part, and especially from that moment, had always taken her mother's side in the frequent arguments with her father, irascible and often drunk, considering her a "victim" who had always suffered the oppression of her husband in order not to deprive her daughter of an assured future.

At the age of 6, her first day at school, at that same village a few miles away, turned out to be far more tolerable than nursery school. In the first place, her mother had continually reassured her during the intervening year, and then, for the first week her mother accompanied her to school, spending the rest of the morning in the village; Sandra thus had time to get to know her teacher and classmates while her mother was still "at hand."

During primary school, the idyllic atmosphere of the preceding period gradually began to break up due to ever more frequent quarrels between her parents over work and the possibility of moving to the city, which her mother was against. During the more intense arguments, Sandra was seized by panic thinking that her mother might die any moment, so that she often eventually felt ill, and the quarrel was then interrupted, usually with her father, overcome by her mother's reproaches, leaving the house, banging the door behind him. Another element which contributed to the break-up of the previous atmosphere were the occasional disagreements between herself and her mother which left her upset, and feeling herself to be the ungrateful daughter. These arguments usually happened when Sandra went to play in her grandmother's garden, leaving her mother alone with the housework. Her mother at first scolded her, warning her about her vivacity and restlessness, and often saying that the only time she had been "good" was when "she had been in her tummy." She then went into a sulk for hours, which to Sandra seemed interminable. One day, when she was 9, during one of these interminable sulks, she felt the impulse to secretly take her father's revolver, slip away again into the garden next door, and aim it at her sleeping grandfather, in order to "test herself" to see whether she was able to control something dangerous.

At the end of primary school, when she was 10, after many arguments, her father got his way and they moved to the city. Seeing the resignation and sadness on her mother's face, Sandra again had the sense of panic that her mother might suddenly die and that she would find herself facing the unknown alone with a father whom she feared. The impact with the city and with middle school was worse than she had imagined in preceding weeks. First of all, she had never seen such a big school with so many teachers and pupils, and this made her feel not a little out of her depth. And then going to school seemed an interminable journey, with traffic jams, tram lines, traffic lights, and so on, all of which often gave her a feeling of some kind of vortex. The first few months in the city were thus months of fear, during which she only felt safe and sheltered in the afternoons at home with her mother. Then, bit by bit, she got to know her teachers and classmates, so that by the end of the year she felt much more at ease.

Sandra remembered quite vividly that morning in class at the age of 12, when she experienced her first menstruation, as menarche had been a tremendous fright for her. She had had no idea what was about to happen to her, given that her mother had not even touched upon "certain" subjects, and she herself had withdrawn whenever she had heard her peers discussing them. When she suddenly realized she was wet with blood, she immediately panicked, afraid she might die at any moment. She took no notice of what her teachers or classmates said and demanded to be taken home immediately to her mother, who was the only person she could trust.

The onset of menstruation changed the dimensions of life in which Sandra had lived up till that point. Her mother, while never touching on delicate subjects, had emphasized the control she should exercise over herself now that she was no longer a child, but Sandra never really understood what should be controlled. Furthermore, her father, who, apart from the arguments with her mother, for years had been a figure absent from family life, had suddenly taken on the role of "sexual controller" of his daughter whom he saw as being lost in the human jungle that he pictured the city to be. As has already been seen in her affective history, there thus began that long period of isolation and continual clashes with her father—a period in which she had been able to experience for herself what it might have meant for her mother to have had to put up with such a man all her life. Thus, every time she managed to escape her father's control by tricking him, she had the sense that she could instead have held her own against him, and in so doing felt she was "redeeming" her mother as well, who had surrendered only for love of Sandra.

Repeatedly passing "through the moviola" the sequence of critical scenes, Sandra arrived at an appreciable reappraisal of her past history as the developmental organization of her phobic meaning gradually became clear to her.

Sandra, although feeling that her perturbing emotions and fears were in some way linked to her relationship with her mother, was not able, however, to glimpse any connection other than the fact that contact with her mother alleviated them. As for the rest, the connecting thread of the whole history consisted of an indirect inhibition of her exploratory behavior and autonomy which was implicitly actuated through the attentions and solicitations of a mother who was, moreover, much loved. It was precisely this indirectness which had made it impossible right from the beginning for Sandra to refer the perturbing experiences to parental behavior and attitudes, nor could she recognize them and appraise them as emotional qualities inherent in her subjective experience.

The memory from when she was 3–4 years old particularly highlighted this aspect if one put into focus this scene and "took seriously" the irritation and anger as the "facts" to be explained, and tried to make her change perspective in seeing them, through a continuous shifting between subjective and objective viewpoints. Thus, while she tried to reconstruct the scene from the outside, trying to insert it in the entire social situation in progress, she recalled how those situations in which the whole village turned out in the fields always became joyous occasions for the children who found they could all play together near the adults who were working. As she was talking about this she fell silent, suddenly realizing how in forcing her to play with the earth dolls which she was patiently making, her mother had managed to keep her near her, making it impossible for her to go and play with the other children. Gradually, after the first few moments of bewilderment, as the scene started to become clear to her in this perspective, Sandra had a strong emotional reaction: visibly anxious and pale, she said she felt faint and wanted to lie down. She recovered after a few minutes and said that for the moment she did not wish to dwell on this episode and wanted instead to be reassured about the moment of "feeling unwell" she had just experienced. From the following session on, however, it was evident that considerable change had come about in her perspective on the past, so that in passing the other significant scenes "through the moviola," she was soon able to trace the same connecting thread which she had suddenly seen during that stressful emotional experience.

Thus, in the episode of the nursery school at the age of 5, she was now in a position to see how the tendency to keep her daughter with her at home had made it possible for her mother to "take literally" what were perhaps the common complaints of a child the first time she goes away from home. In the same way, she now realized that her mother's continual reassurances during the whole year before going to school and her mother's availability in staying near the school, in giving her an assiduous sense of protection also gave her, implicitly, the image of an extremely dangerous world in which being alone meant being defenseless.

Furthermore, it slowly become evident to her that the impossibility of referring perturbing feelings to her mother's behavior had forced them to be experienced as localized in the physical aspects of the self, and this, in turn, had gradually lead to a "sensorial" decoding of any emotional modulation.

Any novelty (school, city, menstruation, etc.) could only be appraised as fear, which had become the most easily recognizable emotional modulation in her range of perceivable emotions. Such sensorial decoding was particularly evident whenever she was struggling with intense sensations deriving from attachment relationships. Thus the fear of suddenly losing a protective base seemed the only way to appraise any possible modification of her mother's availability (clashes with her father, seeing her sad and disheartened when they were moving house, etc.). At the same time, the "feeling unwell" to which such panic attacks frequently gave rise were in perfect harmony with the protective code at home which attributed absolute priority to anything to do with illness (and in fact her feeling unwell instantly put a stop to any quarrel going on at the time).

Passing them repeatedly through the "moviola," those situations appeared particularly important where she felt contrasting feelings in an attachment relationship, such as a threat of "emotional separation" (her mother's sulks, her own fear of distancing herself from her mother, etc.) together with a "sense of constriction" (feeling herself to be at the mercy of her mother's sulks, being constrained to stay near her in order to feel protected, etc.). It was in these circumstances that there emerged both her fear of losing control and the need to test herself in order to control her fear (as exemplified by the episode of the pistol). In this sense, the scene in the fields at the age of 3 or 4 became more and more significant in her eyes, given that it coincided with the first fear of losing control of which she had any trace.

If, from the onset of menstruation, one focused on the whole period of isolation and of the clashes with her father, it became clear to her that taking on the role of the one who redeemed her mother from an unhappy marriage, suffered only because of love for her daughter, was the way of maintaining, although shifting its level, that complicity with her mother which continued to give her a sense of privilege and protection. At the same time, "standing up to her father" had served her as a "bench test" to sharpen her controlling, competitive style which would then emerge fully in her subsequent dealings with men.

Finally, about three quarters of the way through developmental analysis, there occurred another particularly intense emotional situation (although not at the same level as the one that came about while working on her memory of when she was 3–4 years old) which coincided with Sandra's "discovery" of how her mother had probably felt the same fears as she had all her life. Indeed, she suddenly realized that she could recall no circumstances when her mother had been alone at home, or gone somewhere on her own. She clearly recalled, for example, that even during her first week at elementary school when her mother had come with her to the nearby village, she had always brought someone with her (cousin, mother-in-law, or whatever) to avoid being alone in a small village where everyone had known her all her life. This discovery was no small matter for Sandra, as it automatically called into question one of the mainstays of her developmental history, that is: her mother had never left her husband because of love for her daughter. Now it seemed evident that this "putting up with a marriage" was simply the name that her mother had given to her fear of finding herself having to face the world alone. It is interesting to note that as this change in her mother's image was taking place, Sandra seemed in parallel to see the world in a less threatening and alarming way, and indeed at just that time, during a holiday period, she decided to take an intercontinental flight with her husband, while a few months previously, the simple possibility of having to take a plane would have left her in despair.

In the case of Winnie, who was still in a developmental stage, analyzing her past history meant further deepening the self-observational level reached in the preceding work, reconstructing, the organization, over the years, of her way of drawing out a sense of self through the attunement to the perceived expectations of a significant figure.

For Winnie it was her incompetence and lack of will that had made her prefer, for as long as she could remember, to "identify herself" in others. The family was involved insofar as it had always supplied her with a safe, cushioned environment in which her way of doing things could be complied with.

Her family had indeed always been considered a model for the whole neighborhood, both because of her parents' behavior, totally dedicated to work and to their daughters, who lacked for nothing, and also because of the always affectionate and harmonious family atmosphere. Moreover, this had been true since her parents were engaged and passed for a model couple for all the other young people, given the quality and harmony of their affection. Apart from some small disagreements taking place just before the marriage, which she had heard about from other sources, her parents appeared to be a model couple and for their daughters they wished the good fortune of having a marriage like their own.

The very first images of life appear to be fairly toned down and not accompanied by any particular sensations; they concerned the house, the figures of her parents, and a nanny, with whom Winnie remembered she always played with joy and who went away when Winnie was 4.

Two memories that appeared to be of a certain import both went back to the age of 3. The first, before the birth of her sister, was one of her few memories of physical contact with her father, where he, holding her in his arms, continually pretended to throw her in the air. Winnie, having done this before, knew very well that it was a game and laughed blissfully until she saw the worried face of her mother who was looking at her and telling her to stop. Suddenly she felt frightened to death, burst into unrestrainable tears, and wanted to get down. The other memory took place some months after the birth of her sister, whom Winnie had received with joy, thinking of a possible playmate in the games she and Nanny played. One afternoon she was next to her mother who was feeding the baby, and driven by the desire to make herself noticed by her little sister who was intent on her feeding-bottle, she took a chocolate from the table and pretended to give it to her. Her mother inveighed against her, saying that what drove her to do this was the desire to harm her sister because she was wildly jealous of her. Winnie stood as if turned to stone in discovering herself to be so bad and malicious, so much so that she was afraid of herself and did not dare leave her mother, who in the meantime had carried on feeding the baby as if nothing had happened.

At the age of 4, Winnie was a very composed, sensible girl, of whom her mother would talk proudly to friends who came to visit. This was when Nanny had to return to her village, and Winnie was very distressed by it. She remembered, however, that while Nanny embraced her, weeping dreadfully, she was very embarrassed and did not really know what was going on "as grown-ups never cry, and children, when they cry, stop at once."

The rare moments in which she lost a little of her habitual composure were when she complained that her mother never came to fetch her from the nursery, but instead sent a friend whom Winnie had to call Aunty. Winnie wanted to be like the other children, but to her protests her mother promptly replied that she was "an egotist" and "ungrateful," and Winnie, immediately feeling herself to be inadequate, no longer knew for what "real" reason she had made her request.

When she was 5, her maternal grandmother died unexpectedly, and her mother, despite having been very attached to her, dealt with all the necessary details without tears or an atmosphere of grief, so that Winnie was not in the least perturbed by it. The only thing which frightened her to death, so that she burst into tears, losing her habitual control, was seeing her father embracing her mother. This was something not habitual with them and for a moment she had thought that he might harm or even kill her.

On the other hand, while never explicitly saying bad things about him but extolling his virtues as a tireless worker, her mother between the lines tended to negatively redefine her husband's way of being, hinting that she was the model to follow. This had always been clear to Winnie, so that when she was 5, she felt like ice when for Carnival she asked her mother for a "Zorro" costume she really liked, and her mother replied angrily that she did not really like it at all and was only trying to look like her father. At that moment she again felt overcome by a pervasive sense of uncertainty, no longer knowing whether she really liked Zorro or wanted to spite her mother.

Going to school was prepared for with exhaustive recommendations to always be the most polite, the top of the class, and so on, and concluded with her mother personally taking her to school and introducing her to the teacher as if she were a little genius, imploring Winnie not to make her look bad. Thus primary school became torture for Winnie, who had at all costs to be at the top of the class, while all the time she felt on the point of being overwhelmed by the responsibility for not making her mother look bad. Apart from spending all afternoon studying, which for Winnie was a nightmare, she also had to undergo checks on her homework which her mother made at the end of the day, and in which often, heedless of the fact that Winnie knew the material perfectly well, her mother made her rewrite everything again and again until the handwriting was impeccable.

At the end of primary school, Winnie began menstruating for the first time one morning at school and excitedly ran home to tell her mother, sure that she too would be excited and they would celebrate. Winnie started to recount with great emphasis what had happened to her mother, who was doing the ironing. As she slowly realized that her mother had not even raised her eyes from her ironing, she began to feel as if she were turning to stone and fell silent. Her mother, without raising eyes or making any comment, then told her to fetch some more clothes from the kitchen.

It was from then that Winnie dated the emotional distancing and resentment that she began to feel toward her mother and which soon afterwards, at the start of middle school, would lead into the period of dramatic quarrels which we have seen in connection with her affective history.

Passing the affect-laden scenes "through the moviola" several times, Winnie arrived at a reappraisal both of her past history and of her mother's image, reconstructing the developmental organization of her "externally bound" attitude.

As has been seen through the preceding work, Winnie was well aware by now how her relationship with her mother had become a "mirror" for her wherein she could recognize her internal states, but without it being at all clear to her what role her mother as a person might have played in all this. Besides, if the emergence of the early experience of being demarcated from other people had been interfered with from the beginning, any distancing from a significant and intrusive attachment figure became impossible, and the consequent blurred and wavering experiencing of self can only be appraised as something "constitutively" given.

Thus, the first memory, from when she was 3, was taken by Winnie as an example of how her inconsistency and passing from joy to tears on the basis of an opinion expressed by another was something born with her. On the other hand, if this was thoroughly focused on, trying both to make her take up an external viewpoint and to make her differentiate the sense of self from her mother's behavior—seeing the latter in the perspective of *drawing out* an image of her mother as a person—a whole series of new data began to present itself to her. What struck her as most confusing was the reason for which her mother had spoken to her, a 3-year-old, and not to her father, who should have been the natural decision maker as to the running of the family and the upbringing of the children. If one continued to make her focus on this aspect with "eyes of the present," there began to emerge the ambiguity of the communicative style of her family which she was by now beginning to recognize. It now seemed clear to her that her mother, while asserting the opposite, did not in fact consider her husband capable of the role of father, and without explicitly saying so, demanded from Winnie absolute emotional complicity in excluding him from that role—without, moreover, taking into account the mood that her daughter may have been in at that moment. She was able to see that finding herself at the center of a camouflaged and ambiguous situation in which she could take no position was thus what must have thrown her into a panic, rather than any possible danger in the game itself.

On the other hand, focusing on her second memory from when whe was 3, while she was near her mother who was feeding the baby, it seemed clear to Winnie that her mother did not take into account her feelings and intentions but consistently anticipated and redefined them, thus preventing her from developing emotions and opinions on her own. The consequent pervasive sense of indefiniteness and un-reliability in recognizing immediate experiencing eventually made her more reliant on external frames of reference. Thus the scene with Nanny when she was 4 now gave her an image of herself as a child so engaged in adhering to standards of life which had been presented to her that she was incapable of recognizing and appreciating what had surely been one of the most authentic and spontaneous emotional situations of her childhood. In addition, it became ever more clear to her that, as her composure and "sensibleness" increased, in the at-tempt to meet up to her mother's perceived expectations, so the possibility of recognizing spontaneous emotions and attitudes both in herself and in others progressively diminished, as was also illustrated by her reaction to her father who "unexpectedly" embraced her mother.

Given Winnie's young age, hers was a still recent past in which memories retained the vividness and emotional resonance which wanes in adulthood, and as such were easier to reconstruct. Therefore, while one was proceeding with the focusing on childhood (for her, practically "late news"), Winnie was more and more able to recognize, in all the critical scenes, that invariant element which had always characterized her experiencing of her relationship with her mother: that of never having had the sense of being a person unto herself with her own views and emotions. This blurred sense of self (which now made her see in another light her feeling of emptiness and her fear of not being able to feel enough) derived from the way in which she had experienced and appraised the variable combinations of the two basic attitudes that her mother had always had toward her, that is: that of anticipating and redefining her intentions and emotions (the episode of the chocolate, of "Zorro," etc.) and that of the disconfirmation both indirect (making her rewrite her homework, ignoring the fact that she already knew the material) and direct (illustrated by the menstruation episode).

Furthermore, in parallel, Winnie's image of her mother was undergoing modification. Already during the preceding phase of therapy, Winnie no longer believed that her mother was an absolute model of perfection to which she should correspond at all costs. This change in perspective had made her see the "victimizing" attitudes of her mother as "relational tricks" with which to manipulate the members of the family in such a way as to have control of the running of the family. Winnie, however, while understanding that these attitudes of her mother's could not be ends in themselves, had never been able to make out a link with possible existential problems that her mother as a person may have had. During reconstruction of past history, however, it became clearer that, behind the facade, there must be something that was not working with her parents as a couple. The episode when she was 5, when she was frightened at seeing her father embrace her mother, had made her reflect and had emphasized for her that her parents had never had between them even the most trivial affection which is normally seen between couples. The continual negative light in which her father was put and the immediate jealousy her mother showed whenever her daughters expressed tastes or preferences that might give evidence of an attachment to their father, all bore out for her the sensation of a profound schism between them which had never appeared in any visible fashion.

It was then that there suddenly came to mind, with a clarity that astonished her, the rumors that she had heard through other people (cousins, cleaners, etc.) many years before about the "disagreements" her parents had had just before their marriage. Her mother *in extremis,* and to avoid being seen in a bad light by everyone, had succeeded in forcing the father—who was involved with another woman—to give up his plans to call off the wedding. Turning their daughters against him and excluding him from the family without once referring to the fundamental problem was thus what had allowed her mother to not make her defeat explicit and at the same time to take revenge on a man who, having refused her, had felt constrained to face up to the commitments he had made.

Intuiting her mother's secret considerably changed Winnie's attitude toward her; she no longer felt resentment toward her, and instead came to view her as a troubled woman who, in a very simplistic fashion, had attempted to resolve all her problems by selling a perfect image of herself which could not be called into question. It was therefore no longer surprising or upsetting for Winnie to realize that her mother would probably go on all her life criticizing her daughters' eating behavior, romantic affairs, school results, etc., but by now she was sure that this was her mother's problem.

For Gregory, it had always been an effort to "feel worthy" of the abnegation and devotion which his parents had spent on the family and children, forgoing all the other aspects of life. This did not depend on some "latent" rebellion or unwillingness on his part, but rather on the fact that there had always been "something" in him, which could not be precisely defined, but which he had to be on constant guard against.

His parents, fervent Catholics, had always considered religious commitment to be at the center of their lives. The decision to start a family had been for them the equivalent of embracing the religious life, and, as in a convent, everything in the home was subject to rules, prayers, etc., given that religious and moral education of the children (Gregory had a brother 3 years older than he) was the first consideration. Not content, however, with such a commitment, his parents, who were fairly well-off, did all they could in countless benefit and aid activities on religious committees, parish councils, etc. The father, a magistrate, had always been a little absent emotionally from family life, and his presence at home, at least for the children, consisted of philosophical and religious explanations of moral values and of comments on passages from the Bible, which he expected should be known by heart by the children. His mother, a totally uneffusive woman of firm principles—Gregory did not remember one embrace or kiss of hers—until the eve of the wedding had been undecided as to whether she should become a nun, and had always considered the condition of married woman as an expedient renunciation of a superior spiritual life. With the children, she therefore had an attitude which more or less ran like this: "I have forgone sainthood in order to live with you; you must repay me for this by being stainless and without sin."

The first images of life concerned, on the one hand, playing alone in various parts of the house, accompanied by a sense of serenity and tranquility; on the other, they concerned his mother who, meteor-like, would every so often interrupt his games (because they were noisy, because it was prayer time, etc.), leaving Gregory with a feeling of personal "unpleasantness" which stayed with him for a long time. Of this period (about the age of 3) he remembered a particular occasion, perhaps the only one, in which his mother, instead of interrupting him as usual, started to play with him. Gregory for the moment was astonished beyond words, but did not have to time to feel content, as he suddenly felt as if he were being "made fun of" and this immediately produced that same sense of unpleasantness, which made him stop playing despite his mother's insistence that they continue. The occasions of greater contact with his mother when he was 3 or 4 were in early afternoon, when she withdrew with him to tell him stories from the Bible, adapted as fables; in these circumstances, Gregory again felt, after the first few minutes, an unexpected sense of irritation which immediately became transformed into that unpleasant sense of self, which lasted for most of the afternoon. Gregory was not sent to nursery school because it was considered superfluous, and he therefore spent most of his time at home with his mother, as his brother was at school most of the day; however, his mother was always busy and spent the minimum amount of time with him necessary for ethical and religious education. Gregory had always experienced this period in a somewhat contrasting fashion, given that, on the one hand, he felt so alone that "time never passed," but, on the other, he did not have the freedom of movement of a child alone because he felt he was always in his mother's "sight"; she, although busy, did not let him out of her sight for a moment and was ever ready to call him to her.

About the age of 4 or 5, there was a significant memory because, among other reasons, it featured his father. Gregory had been absolutely forbidden to look out of the window, even though there was no particular cause for alarm as they lived almost at ground level, and the windows, too high for him to reach, were also barred. One afternoon, trusting perhaps in a moment's "inattention" on the part of his father, who was in the living room with him, Gregory looked out for a moment to watch the children playing in the courtyard underneath, which, despite all the warnings, had always held a great attraction for him. His father jumped out of his armchair, and with a riding-whip in hand, followed him all around the living room until, in a corner and under the threat of the whip, Gregory had to kneel and recite a *mea culpa* on the misdeed in front of the family, who had in the meantime rushed in. This moral punishment or "humiliation" (as Gregory called it) seemed to be the essential ingredient in the upbringing strategy of his father who missed no chance to administer it, both to him and to his brother, as a reaction to transgressions which often appeared negligible even to an unindulgent eye, such as his mother's.

To the age of 5 there belongs a memory that was meaningful to Gregory as it represented the first time that there emerged what he called the "doubt of the solipsism" which had for some years frightened him very much. It was perhaps the first time he had been alone in the courtyard underneath and looked at the trees and the people at the windows. Suddenly he had the powerful sensation that everything he could see—including other people and himself—might be just an image in his mind, that is, an invention which did not correspond to reality. The sense of bewilderment and panic was so intense that it drove him immediately back into the house under the watchful eye of his mother.

Although long looked forward to, the first day at school at the age of 6 turned out to be a somewhat disconcerting experience. As the school was only a few hundred meters away, Gregory, after the usual countless warnings, was sent to school alone, and as soon as he arrived had a moment of complete disorientation and "felt lost" in the midst of so many children. He recovered after a moment, but could not understand the mechanism by which children were assigned to classes, and so, in accordance with his logic of the moment, he joined a class which had just formed. The result was that for the rest of the morning he wandered from class to class and at a certain point wondered if there was any end to them; when finally he managed to find the class he was assigned to, thanks to the intervention of teachers and janitors, he found himself feeling quite lost and a little ashamed in the midst of his classmates who had already got to know each other and who looked at him amusedly. This theme of shame and feeling lost in class and at school remained a constant for the whole time Gregory was at primary school, and only gradually began to fade with the beginning of middle school. Indeed, up to the age of 11, he had been obliged to wear his elder brother's clothes, and this, added to his feeling awkward in group situations and clumsy at games, accentuated his sense of personal unpleasantness.

At primary school, Gregory was a sensible child, more mature than his age, and although he still felt awkward with his classmates, he was much respected by them and admired for his knowledge and scholastic performance. However, as he matured and his moral education became more rigid and intransigent, the norms and prohibitions multiplied, but so did the capability for more autonomous reasoning and the possibilities for amusement (cinema, television, peers, etc.), with the result that his doubts also multiplied as to what was sin and what was not. When he was 7 or 8, these doubts often tormented him in the afternoons while he was studying in his room, to the point where he at times felt a sense of being a despicable person who would swear just for the pleasure of doing so. At this point, there appeared in his mind, as on a screen, a phrase so vulgarly blasphemous that it terrified him; however, he immediately worked out the system of adding a question mark to the phrase the moment it appeared, and immediately afterwards would loudly reply inside himself, "No! No!"

These religious dilemmas, even though accompanied by frequent confessions to the priest, remained more or less under control during primary school and the beginning of middle school, until, at the beginning of his last year at middle school, they started to intensify progressively. Already the passage to middle school, where he had found himself in mixed classes for the first time, had perturbed and disoriented him not a little, revealing to him the existence of sensations and impulses he knew nothing about. To this was added the discovery of masturbation which perturbed and upset him even more.

One afternoon, at the age of 13, he was talking, perhaps a little distractedly, to his mother and in gesticulating inadvertently touched one of her breasts. His mother instantly struck him a sound blow, crushed him with a contemptuous look, and hissing "filthy pig" at him, went indignantly back to the kitchen and did not speak to him for 2 weeks. Gregory was instantly sure that he was absolutely unable to control those sensations and impulses which he already mistrusted, and felt with an almost uncontrollable anguish a nullifying sense of personal despicableness. For over 2 years, the need to continually test and retest himself about his moral scruples became more frequent and tormenting. He locked himself away for hours, forcing himself into a self-analysis as exhausting as it was insufficient, so that it finished by his going to confession every day, despite the priest's attempts to dissuade him.

From the age of 15–16 on, Gregory seemed to establish an equilibrium through an almost "ascetic" ethical and moral commitment which had allowed him to avoid all possible opportunities for amusement that might evoke unforeseen sensations and emotions. As will be remembered, this was the period leading up to his first romantic experience, which took place, in fact, the first time that he had decided to loosen the "monk-like" constraints he had been placing on himself for some time.

The individual scenes were passed "through the moviola" several times, and, because of Gregory's acquired ability to differentiate experiencing and explaining, as well as that of reconstructing the multifaceted aspects of feelings by shifting alternately between subjective and objective viewpoints, it was possible to reconstruct the developmental organization of his obsessive meaning, while reordering at the same time his view of the past.

As we have seen, ambivalent patterns of attachment—where an explicit facade of absolute devotion and concern was simultaneously intertwined with implicit rejecting attitudes—had been, from the beginning, an integral part of the perceived existential situation. In this way, it had always been nearly impossible for Gregory to refer to the attitude of his parents the consequent antithetical feelings about himself, so that these could only be experienced as something that was part of him. In focusing, therefore, the key point consisted precisely of taking this perturbing sense of unpleasantness of himself not as "something given" but as a "fact" that had to be explained, and thus find a different perspective with which to look at the critical scenes by shifting continuously between different self-observational viewpoints.

As he began to put into focus, in this way, the images of his relationship with his mother during his preschool years, Gregory easily realized that his oscillations between opposing feelings (serenity/ tranquility vs. annoyance/irritation) were constantly correlated with experiencing his mother's attitude as "available"—she was always with him ("She likes me/I'm a 'positive' boy")—and simultaneously as "not available"—she was noneffusive and inattentive to his feelings and needs ("She dislikes me/I'm a 'negative' boy"). In particular, the memory from when he was 3, when she started to play with him, turned out to be highly significant in clarifying this aspect for him. In fact, his wonder at her availability was immediately mismatched by the perception of her total lack of spontaneity in playing with him, triggering anger and hostility feelings ("she's just making fun of me") which could have been appraised only as a pervasive unacceptability of his way of being (e.g., his sense of personal unpleasantness). It is important to emphasize that seeing himself and his mother in this perspective evoked a notable emotional activation in Gregory. He noticed this himself from his attitude, more controlled and embarrassed than usual, and from the need he often had to clarify (to the therapist and to himself) that none of this excluded his continuing to feel "positive" sentiments toward his mother.

The episode with his father, occurring when he was 4 or 5, while showing him another variant of the same kind of ambivalent attachment, also made clear for him that the demand for obedience actually corresponded to a request for an absolute, unconditional adherence to norms to be respected as such (being forbidden to look out of the window, which had nothing to do with concrete reasons of safety); the absoluteness of the request excluded any curiosity and impulsiveness, so that any transgression was punished by the "nullifying" of any spontaneous behavior so typical for children ("humiliation"). Moreover, it seemed ever more evident to him that his parents had always considered him a "miniature adult," holding superfluous what for a child is indispensable, such as contact with peers—the ban on taking part in their games in the courtyard, the decision not to send him to nursery school, etc.—to the point of requiring from him behavior beyond the ability of a child of his age (how to orient oneself alone in the confusion of the first day at school).

Of particular importance was the episode that occurred when he was 5, during which there surfaced the "solipsistic doubt" which Gregory had always seen as a brilliant example of the fact that there was something in him which had to be guarded against. As he repeatedly focused on the scene from an objective viewpoint (with both the eyes of the past and those of the present), he was able to notice that intense sensations of bewilderment and panic were the way in which he appraised an ambivalent and antithetical sense of self. That is, the structuring of a psychophysiological modulation characterized by abrupt and recurrent oscillations between opposing feelings went in parallel with the emergence of split patterns of self-recognition which, being mutually exclusive, interfered with a unitary self-experiencing.

It then began to be clear to him that the only way of controlling the ambivalence of his subjective experiencing had been to prioritize the emerging possibilities offered by concrete cognitive abilities, which as well as facilitating the adherence to ethical norms, also seemed to guarantee him a nonambivalent understanding. Already in the episode of his first day at school, at the age of 6, it was evident that his selective inattention to the emotional modulation provided by immediate experiencing (need for help and support by adults present) led him to trust that "reasoning"—he should have been able to find the class by himself. Thus, as he slowly managed to control the ongoing emotional modulation to the point where he could exclude it, the contrasting and ambivalent feelings which his parental upbringing evoked in him became appraisable only as doubts which called into question his adherence to an order of absolute rules, and thus the acceptability of his sense of self.

It was precisely his adherence to rationality and logic that enabled him to avoid those intolerable sensations of disunity and inconsistency (the "solipsistic doubts") given that the application in his tests and retests of the "all-or-nothing" procedure ("If I am not impeccable then I am surely despicable") guaranteed that he felt a unitary and consistent sense of self, whether positive or negative. The expedient of putting a question mark at the end of the blasphemous phrase—so that an affirmation became a "hypothetical" question—made him smile with something between amusement and embarrassment as he was reflecting on it while viewing it in slow motion. It was clearer and clearer to him, in fact, that, already at that time, his rationality was based almost exclusively on the pure and simple formal adherence to logical procedures, rather than on the consistency of the contents.

Finally, putting into focus the scene from when he was 13, it became evident to him that in that afternoon the behavior of his mother had confirmed for him, with no hope of appeal, what he had always perceived in the relationship with her: that he was capable of being so unworthy and despicable as to disappoint and cause suffering to precisely those people who had dedicated their lives to him. The succeeding 2 years spent in tests and retests, even in their limiting pervasiveness, helped him to find an equilibrium which at first seemed impossible. Shutting himself up in his room among his books, and his devotion in church, were admired at home, and this made him feel less criticized and hence less despicable; in addition, his exaggerated control of even the most banal "suspicious" sensations had progressively refined for him the procedure of perceiving an acceptable sense of self through the more or less complete exclusion of his emotional life. However, the ascetic, isolated life arrived at in this way was held in a somewhat precarious balance, inevitably destined to topple the moment he started a sentimental career. As we have seen, having to test and retest every sensation that an engagement evoked in him in order to be sure of the quality and rightness of his feelings, as well as calling into question that acceptability of the self at which he had arrived after so much effort, would also eventually result in a series of disappointments and anxieties in his romantic relationships.

FINAL CONSIDERATIONS

In contrast to the preceding phases, in which one is working on experiences which—being current or originating for the most part in the recent past—are more vivid and richer in detail and thus more easily reconstructible, in a developmental analysis, one is working with much vaguer material, poor in detail, and, above all, experienced much more as something taken absolutely for granted and not deserving, therefore, any further reflection and explanation. We are thus dealing with a somewhat more exacting phase, both for the therapist, who must have a certain ability in assessing critical memories and in setting the self-observational contexts capable of being reordered, and for the client, who finds him- or herself in the particular emotional condition of experiencing a changing perspective toward emotional schemata and cognitive patterns closely interwoven with his or her sense of continuity and sameness.

Making clients repeatedly go back and forth throughout their developmental history is, undoubtedly, the self-observational process that triggers the most important reordering of critical immediate experiences. This process results in a reframing of the memory of those events and also a high level of distancing and decentering from recurrent affective tonalities which are an integral part of ongoing patterns of self-perception. It is moreover possible to distinguish different structural levels of memory reframing from equally different levels of reordering and emotional activation.

A first level of reframing consists of attaining a more exhaustive comprehension of a vague but intriguing memory, with no concomitant change in the perspective with which the scene is currently perceived. In other words, there is a reordering of data *within the same frame* which allows a better focusing on a whole series of details, but which leaves the affective tonality triggered by the scene unaltered. This is the type of reframing that comes about most commonly during developmental analysis, the utility of which essentially lies in facilitating the reframings of a higher level; they do not otherwise have a remarkable therapeutic value.

A second type of reframing results from a change in the perspective endorsed on a scene up to that point; it consists of a reordering of *the whole memory frame* which makes possible the emergence of new data; it is matched by a reorganization of the affective tonality usually triggered by the scene. This is what happened with Richard's memory from the age of 4 when his father was worried about providing for him; that of Sandra when she was 3 or 4 about the earth dolls her mother made; Winnie's memory from age 3 when her father played at pretending to throw her in the air; and so on. We are dealing with a type of reframing which is notably effective therapeutically and which is almost invariably accompanied by a fairly considerable emotional activation, as exemplified by Sandra's reaction as she focused on the scene of the earth dolls.

A third type of reframing results from *the recombination between whole sets* of already reordered memory frames which makes possible the emergence of aspects of self and of one's own past of which clients are totally unaware. This is what happened when Richard suddenly realized that his father had "never sought him out"; when Sandra "discovered" the similarity between her fears and her mother's; when Winnie intuited the "secret" that her mother had always tried to hide. This is the most effective kind of reframing for proceeding with that modification of viewpoint of oneself that the client began at the start of developmental analysis.

The emotional modulation continuously provided both by going back and forth through the past and also by reframing processes triggers a parallel reordering of basic effective themes, in which the increased distancing from critical emotional dimensions is matched by their recombination with the new tonalities of the feelings which have emerged (*third level* of emotional restructuring).

One may therefore say that at the developmental level, the change in the "Me" appraisal of the "I" consists of shifting from experiencing one's praxis of living as something "given" to appraising it as the basic, self-organized pattern of coherence that consistently orders past and present experiences in such a way that a recognizable continuity results. Hence, with the change that comes about during the first half of the second phase, emotional disturbances, rather than as "given," are appraised as "co-products" of one's way of experiencing affect. With the change that takes place at the end of the second half, the same thing happens for the affective style, the recognized coherence of which is increasingly experienced as the unfolding of one's personal meaning. With developmental analysis, what is no longer taken for granted is exactly that personal meaning which comes to be experienced as the lifelong process of scaffolding the coherence of one's being-in-the-world.

As developmental analysis is gradually reaching completion, the therapist begins to prepare the setting with which to conclude the therapeutic work carried out. Usually the aspects which one needs to deal with in this preparatory work are the following:

The client's greater awareness of his or her own level of functioning reached by changing the viewpoint of oneself and one's own history is invariably accompanied by a whole series of contrasting emotions which give rise to a fairly typical sense of ambiguity. On the one hand, he or she feels a sense of security deriving from experiencing oneself as the active protagonist of one's own praxis of living; on the other, however, he or she also feels a sense of disappointment deriving from feeling that one's praxis of living, as it was being defined step by step, came out differently from what was expected. In other words, if at the beginning of therapy all the problems depended on the fact that one does not know who one is, at the end the main problem becomes precisely that one does know.

Clients at this stage, even though in different ways and with different expressions, show a certain intolerance toward their own way of being, which often comes to be experienced as the source of all future problems. Rather than trying to guess, "shooting in the dark," or developing forecasts of varying degrees of detail from which to derive rules of behavior to be applied, the most efficacious method for dealing with this stage is to allow the client to put into focus the dynamics and coherence of his or her personal meaning through other viewpoints, beyond that which seems to be perturbing at the moment. Thus, if in running over the connecting thread of the whole past history, one reconstructs how through it the client has nevertheless managed to transform difficult existential conditions into situations of personal growth, it becomes possible to highlight the idea that the orthogenetic directionality of a developmental pathway corresponds simply to a generative and original way of ordering experience.

Right from the opening exchanges, moreover, the therapist, both with the self-observational method and his or her personal attitudes and behavior, has always given particular care to construing and developing the viewpoint which says that there is no objective, unequivocal mode of organizing experience which can be identified as "valid" as opposed to "erroneous." The client then begins to notice that his or her personal meaning is both the necessary constraint for "having-a-world" and also corresponds at the same time to his or her degree of liberty in that world, given that it defines neither the possible ways of "being-in-it" nor the forms which experience may assume through them. This is what Saint-Exupéry (1942/1979) meant many years ago when he said, in his simple and direct style, that "freedom and constraint are two aspects of the same necessity, the necessity of being the man you are and not another. You are free to be that man, but not another."

Thus, a "depressive" personal meaning simply brings forth a possible world in which the experience of loss is the generative dimension for discovering cognitive and emotional domains, without defining whether, in unfolding such a dimension, the subject will become, for example, an original writer with an intense and full emotional life or whether he or she will become a drunk, of varying degrees of desperation, who will spend his or her days in solitude. It will now seem more and more evident that one's own way of being, rather than an inescapable existential situation, is instead the inescapable underlying condition for structuring a variety of possible existential dimensions.

As it becomes clear that the exploratory work undertaken together is drawing to a conclusion, the therapist should gradually construct a setting for preparing and facilitating the client's disengagement from the therapeutic context.

"Technically" speaking, the problem consists of transforming the therapeutic relationship into one of supervision, as if the client were a fledgling therapist who occasionally submits to a more expert colleague the developments of the case being followed, with the sole difference that the case under consideration is the client's own. In this way, the sessions begin to progressively thin out, becoming one every 2 months, one every 3 or 4 months, and so on, until they stop completely, just as in the case of a therapist under supervision who at a certain point feels able to continue alone. This kind of procedure does not usually create any important difficulties. Firstly, most clients have already realized that the therapeutic work has reached its culmination, beyond which it would become more and more repetitive, and, secondly, the "self-observational training" followed during the therapy has implicitly prepared the client for the role of "therapist under supervision" and thus he or she is not at all surprised when the moment comes to take on this role explicitly.

However, even though it has been prepared and facilitated in this way, it should be remembered that a disengagement from a therapeutic context still corresponds to an emotional separation within an interpersonal relationship which has for a long time held two people in close contact. It is therefore almost inevitable that at this stage there should emerge, more or less explicitly, a series of emotions (an alternation of opposing and collaborative attitudes, etc.) which are an integral part of the way in which emotional detachments or separations are developed (see Chapter 4). Rather than taking them as "resistances" and simply attempting to diminish their scope, the therapist should instead use them, both in order to clarify further aspects of the client's bonding style, as well as to renegotiate the reciprocal roles and the relational rules their relationship will follow while the current transformation proceeds.

APPENDIX: GUIDELINES FOR THE RECONSTRUCTION OF A DEVELOPMENTAL HISTORY

• Preliminary gathering of data concerning family structure at the moment of birth (members, ages, jobs).
• Profile of mother and father as individual "characters" (attitudes, emotional temperament, hobbies, social skills, roles in the family) and as a "couple" (how parents and sociofamilial network tell how they met, the engagement, level of openness and mutual support between parents, etc.).

The aim of a developmental history is to reconstruct the sequences of crucial events that have given rise to the opinions, explanations, and meanings to which the client refers when recounting a given period of his or her past history. As a useful general method, begin with a general reconstruction of the course of life in the corresponding developmental period, and then proceed to focus on specific domains. Within each domain there should then be identified the affect-laden events that deserve reconstruction and re-ordering in the moviola setting. The areas of inquiry within each developmental state that merit exploration in depth are, in broad outline, the following:

Infancy and Preschool Years (0–6 Years Old)

Detailed Gathering of Earliest Available Memories

• Focus on how parents are depicted, other family members, the home, the outside world, etc.
• Detailed focus on the emotional tonalities connected to each image.

Reconstruction of the Course of Family Life
in the Preschool Period

• Degree of presence/absence of parental figures, type of emotional atmosphere generated by their presence or absence, usual attitudes of parents (such as the level of effusion and emotional support which could be expected from them, types of warnings and advice, rules and restrictions, etc., that were transmitted explicitly and implicitly by their attitudes and behavior).
• What kind of child people said the client was, and what sense of self this provoked; what games, stories, or fairy tales were favorites.
• Type of participation and role the family had in the social network (how being with others was presented; opportunities, or otherwise, of spending time with other children, etc.). Type of family reaction to concurrent events (loss, separation, moving house, money problems, etc.).

Quality of Emotional Reciprocity and Attachment in the
Relationship with Each Parent Reconstructable through
Affect-Laden Interactions with Them

• Predictability and control on the child's part during affect-laden interactions with parent.
• Feeling tones and emotions evoked in affect-laden interactions with parent and the modality with which it was possible to express them.
• Type of immediate experiencing of self accompanying those feeling tones and emotions.
• Development of exploratory behavior and the ability to cope with transitory separations when going off to nursery school and at the beginning of primary school (reactions to detachment from the home, to the presence of other children and of teachers, etc.).

Childhood (6–11 Years Old)

Reconstruction of the Child's Life Structure during
Elementary School

• At school: Relationship with children of the same age and the role taken in class and in the broader school group. Progress of scholastic performance and any ups and downs it may have suffered during the elementary stage.

• In the family: How the typical week went, organization of free time (games with parents, other children, etc.) and of time given over to study and to adherence to the norms of upbringing and family routine.

• Attitude of parents toward scholastic performance (expectations, attributions of success or failure, etc.) and toward norms and values to be respected, expressed both directly (through advice and warnings, incentives, chidings, etc.) and indirectly (by describing the merits and demerits of other children of the same age and of other people).

• Attitude of parents and repercussions in family life in the face of concurrent events such as separation, death in the family, money problems, and marriage crises.

Emotional Reciprocity and the Quality of Attachment

• Reconstruction of the parents' image perceived by the child through either "direct" (analysis of affect-laden interactions with the father or mother) or "indirect" (how the father or mother is described when he or she is absent; quality of mother–father relationship; parents' observable interaction with the family's social network) data.

• Reconstruction of the relationship between parents' expectations expressed as strategies of upbringing, effusive attitudes, etc. ("how one felt seen through their eyes") and the child's expectations expressed by taking stances, oppositional attitudes and behavior, demands for autonomy, etc. ("how the child would have liked to be seen by them"); the effect that such a relationship had on the child's immediate experiencing of self.

Early Adolescence and Puberty (11–14/15 Years Old)

Reconstruction of the Modifications in Life Structure
Resulting from Environmental and Maturational Changes

• Going on to middle school and consequent changes in the demands of the scholastic and familial network.

• Pubertal maturation and psychosexual development (bodily transformation and acceptability of own image, attitude to sexuality, place in own age group, etc.).

Influence of Family Attachment on the Ongoing
Self-Reorganization

• Quality of the relationship with the parent of the same sex and his or her readiness to serve as a possible model of adulthood linked to his or her own gender role.

• Quality of the relationship with the parent of the opposite sex and his or her readiness to serve as a "bench test" in appraising the lovableness of one's sexual role.

• Reorganization of family attachment after sexual maturation and any modifications in the perceived images of parents.

Late Adolescence and Youth (15–20 Years Old)

Reconstruction of the Cognitive-Emotional Separation from Parents

• Main experiential domains in which "emotional separation" from parents was followed through, that is, "knowledge dimension" (cultural, political, etc.) and "emotional dimension" (identification with peer group, first love affair, etc.).

• Reconstruction of the oscillations between emotional separation (affirmations of autonomy) and emotional reapproach (demands for protection, recognition, etc.).

Relativization of Parents' Images and Its Effects on the Experience and Appraisal of Self

• Structure and attribution of the perceived change of parents' images (disappointment, lack of protection, loss, etc.).

• Self-referring and appraising the perceived change of attachment figures (self-competence and lovableness, self-esteem and life-programming, etc.).

9

Concluding Remarks

The major obstacle in promoting the advancement of psychotherapy as a science can be traced to the prevalent trend of considering both clinical research and therapeutic work as exclusively "applied" fields quite distinct from basic theoretical work (Forsyth & Strong, 1986; Glasser, 1982; Lambert, 1989; Sommer, 1982; Stone, 1984). However, this distinction between basic and applied research, according to which the former deals with "theory" and the latter with "facts," has been losing value in recent years as people have realized that every observation is a process of differentiation of "events" from a background of *a priori* hypotheses and assumptions and, consequently, that "without theory there are no observable facts" (Lakatos, 1974; Popper, 1972, 1982; Weimer, 1979). It has thus become evident that applied research is none other than a method for advancing that same theoretical research which is the basis for any progress in scientific knowledge.

This disconnection from basic theorizing has meant that therapists have long been too technologically oriented, as if testing and validating a set of techniques were the only "serious" occupation for a clinical psychologist. The ensuing identification of "therapy" with "technique," which tacitly stems from this belief, has inevitably rendered psychotherapeutic research theoretically simplistic and situationally bound. First, the emphasis on application has encouraged therapists to look for immediate relevance to their testing in their available data, consequently neglecting important theoretical constructions set forth by convergent disciplines (evolutionary epistemology, systems theory, etc.). Second, their testing methods have focused only on the immediate therapeutic setting, in attempting to answer the question: "Does technique X work better than technique Y?" thus considering only limited aspects of attitudes, cognitive abilities, and emotional processing.

If asked for an opinion regarding their scant interest in theory, therapists generally protect themselves by saying that theories are of no use to their clients; this would seem obvious, given that the latter have other interests at stake and other work to do. The problem, in actual fact, is that theories assist therapists in setting what the client says or feels within the broader dimension of human experience, and hence also in allowing the planning of an intervention which is neither tritely reassuring nor pretentiously pedagogic.

This situation has resulted in an ever-widening gap between the simplistic concepts therapists hold regarding human behavior (hedonistic determinism, rational supremacy, etc.) and the complexity of the existential crises that their clients portray, with the result that the former are not able to heed the contrasting and multifaceted subjective experiencing brought to them by the latter.

As we have attempted to outline in the first part of this work, the point of departure of any consistent psychological theorizing should be this: understanding is not separable from human existence, so that to exist means literally to know. Hence, rather than being the "impartial" process of representing a "given" reality more or less validly, knowing is the ontological process of constructing a world able to make the ongoing experience of the ordering subject consistent.

If it were clearer that humans are not "philosophers" driven by the desire to find, in any fashion, a "valid" truth, one would perhaps be less astounded by the contrasting, ambiguous feelings with which humans experience the increasing complexity of self-awareness which they come up against during their lifespan. Knowing oneself, indeed, essentially means being able to manage the effect derived from being oneself in the face of the growing clarity with which one perceives the irreversibility of one's own life, and this brings with it the activation of complex emotions (ambiguity, sense of the absurd, etc.) which, although not found in clinical psychology textbooks, are nonetheless essential ingredients of present human experience. The inversion of perspective brought about by seeing consciousness from the viewpoint of he or she who possesses it is well expressed in the following aphorism of Cioran (1981), which is, as usual, most incisive:

"What is truth?" is a fundamental question. But it becomes of little moment compared to the other question: "How can life be borne?" Yet even this pales into insignificance when placed side by side with: "How is one to bear *oneself*?" Here is the key question, to which no one is able to give us an answer. (p. 145)

However vividly and urgently he or she may feel it, not even a therapist is able to supply any conclusive response to that kind of question; it is important, however, that he or she is able to trace what the client experiences as a life-limiting idiosyncracy back to a fundamental theme of our praxis of living, highlighting the fact that the insolubility of this dilemma is part of the essential tension with which we experience selfhood, and which constantly urges us beyond the horizon of our immediate personal experience. Thus, instead of hastily disposing of a seemingly "irrational" question, given the insolubility of the answer, and leaving the client alone with his or her existential anguish, the therapist may share it. By participating in it and intensifying the quality of reciprocal involvement with the client, the therapist assumes an emotional stance implicitly showing that solidarity and affective cohesion between people may together constitute a way of being able to coexist with the dilemma of our existence.

If, furthermore, we consider that, like all primates, our existence unfolds within an intersubjective dimension, and that we can thus only know ourselves in relation to others, the centrality that love and affectivity have in human experience becomes obvious. On the one hand, given that the trends of attachment relationships regulate right from the start the intensity and quality of other emotions (fear, anger, etc.) which modulate their approach–avoidance dynamics, love and affectivity become the central "organizers" of the individual's way of self-experiencing and self-referring (lovableness, self-esteem, etc.). And, given the regulatory role that a significant other's image exerts on ongoing patterns of self-perception, love and affectivity maintain their central role throughout lifespan by scaffolding the relevance of life events and by triggering life crises, and consequent reorganization of personal experience.

Finally, both the ontological nature of knowing and the central role exerted by love and affectivity should become part of a systems/process-oriented approach to the development of different patterns of meaning dimensions (P.M.Orgs.). Indeed, if ontologically the human way of being-in-the-world is by seeking and creating meaning (cf. Smith, 1978a, 1985), then it is possible—within the intersubjective dimension constraining the invariance of human experience—to identify a set of different personal meaning dimensions, in the same way, as it were, that it is possible to identify different physical constitutions within the morphological invariance of the human body. An ontological approach to personality and psychopathology ought to lead to a "science of personal meaning" with an inherent grammar of composition and recombination which will allow us to set out the different patterns of organized coherence that people exhibit in their search for meaning. This is absolutely not another way of pigeonholing the client with a static "diagnostic label" right from the start, as is the case when adopting the descriptive nosography endorsed by the DSM-III-R, that is, when using the lists of critical beliefs supposed to be specific of anxiety, depression, etc. Quite the contrary, adherence to a process-oriented model of personal meaning development, rendering the therapist less externally bound to actual problems, would instead allow him or her to use them in order to foster new levels of comprehension, thus allowing the client's self-organizing processes to influence the therapeutic strategy.

Adopting less technical language than that used in the theoretical section, and closer to that used in everyday work with clients, in the clinical framework of the second part of this book we have tried to exemplify how a cognitive therapy can be nonpersuasive and situationally bound to the attainment of self-control to the extent to which it can construct a strategy of intervention on the basis of more complex theorizing about human functioning. In concluding these notes, we think it will be helpful to take particular notice of two aspects:

The framework presented *is not a technique;* rather it *is a strategy* whose therapeutic efficacy is founded on an explanatory principle of human functioning—that is, on increasing clients' flexibility in assuming alternately different points of view of themselves through the self-observation method, bringing about a parallel increase in levels of self-complexity matched by a more adequate self-appraisal and decoding of immediate experience (Lane & Schwarz, 1987; Linville, 1985, 1987; Markus & Nurius, 1986; Rosenberg & Gara, 1985).

Apart from the exposition of the essential aspects of the self-observation method, we do not think it appropriate to illustrate "techniques" in order to demonstrate the rationale, to guide the client in going back and forth in slow motion, etc. In the first place, all this, apart from being of little help, might give the misleading impression that it is a presentation of yet another set of therapeutic techniques whose efficacy has to be proved. Secondly, a systems/process-oriented therapist does not consider the achievement of a change in the client's viewpoint on him- or herself as a matter of choosing a set of specific techniques; on the contrary, the therapist is free to use any technique, whether already existing or invented on the spot, which allows him or her to develop the strategy of increasing the client's self-flexibility. In other words, as Mahoney succinctly put it several years ago:

> . . . techniques are ritualized methods of communication which ac-
> quire different meanings depending on their derivative contexts. . . . If
> one views the search for increasingly effective techniques as basically
> one of identifying more powerful messengers, one may begin to wonder
> whether contemporary clinical research has begun to confuse the
> message with the messenger. The gist of this last point is that tech-
> niques might be more adequately construed as tools subservient to a
> larger and more elusive endeavor. They offer a valuable assistance in
> structuring and communicating some therapeutic messages, but they
> should not be confused with the latter. (1981, pp. 269–270)

To carry on a process-oriented strategy, both the construction of an adequate emotional context and proper timing are essential.

The construction of an interpersonal setting endowed with an adequate level of emotional involvement essentially depends on how far the therapist is prepared to forgo a guarantee of "objectivity" and of being able to provide the correct and definitive response to every one of the client's questions. Even if not supported by consistent scientific arguments, such pedagogic behavior turns out to be somewhat per-sistent even in therapists who seek to follow nonpersuasive methods precisely because, by limiting emotional involvement, the therapist feels more protected, as is well emphasized in this well-known passage from Gadamer:

> The claim to understand the other person in advance performs the
> function of keeping the claim of the other person at a distance. We are
> familiar with this from the educative relationship, an authoritative
> form of welfare work. (1979, p. 323)

The story turns out quite differently the moment the therapist abandons the role of the outside objective observer and accepts the idea that any knowledge is "participatory" and based on the reciprocal negotiation of a mutual agreement rather than on a mere transmission of data. While he or she will inevitably become more involved in construing the therapeutic setting, the therapist will at the same time become even more aware of the influence that his or her emotional aspects exert on the course of the relationship, and, therefore, on the definition of therapeutic reality itself. That is, the therapist is forced to take into account his or her own emotional oscillations which accompany and modulate his or her ongoing perception and understanding of the client's problem. But such oscillations, though triggered by the interaction with the client, inform not so much about the latter's functioning as about the therapist him- or herself. In other words, as therapists renounce the role of "trustees of objectivity" and enter into the game of self-referentiality, then behind any order they perceive, they cannot but grasp the contour of their own image, and this, besides enhancing self-awareness, also enhances their involvement in the relationship.

Finally, a process-oriented strategy is a progressive, step-like ascension in levels of ordering experience which are more and more structured and integrated, and it is thus essential that in order to be effective it should progress in accordance with proper timing; that is, before proceeding to the construction of a new level of self-observation and self-ordering, the therapist must be sure that the client has achieved stability at the preceding level. Let us take as an example the developmental history, even though the same argument also applies to preceding stages; the client's ability in focusing on the past from a new level of self-appraisal and self-referring interwoven with the growing awareness of his or her functioning is the crucial variable allowing the reconstruction of the past to be carried out with an appreciable level of reordering. In other words, if one were not able to use as a fulcrum the fact that the client already has another point of view of him- or herself, one would arrive at a mere "biographical account" rather than at a developmental analysis, which would not just be useless but actually harmful, because it would inevitably end up by confirming and legitimizing the habitual version endorsed by the client.

The emphasis given to the role that awareness plays in the progress and quality of transformations taking place during lifespan may give rise to the question of whether this emphasis substantially corresponds to making awareness the legitimate heir of rationality.

This in turn would correspond, in practice, to a therapeutic attitude characterized by the excessive induction of awareness as such, proposed as a panacea. If nothing else, this is at least a possible "right way" of bringing one back to oneself. Forgoing the role of impartial, "objective" observer, together with a methodology of system/process investigation, allows us to dispel this doubt, bringing to light the way in which awareness is linked to a whole series of problems.

In the first place, the detailed analysis of the modifications of the level of awareness triggered by a therapeutic setting of this kind makes it clear that awareness is simply *one* of the ways in which a system constructs an image of itself in order to increase the viability of its ordering processes. This image is regulated by the same auto-referential logic on which the whole system is based (i.e., personal meaning) and hence does not correspond to a "right" or "true" image of the self—indicative, that is, of that which the system is in itself—but rather to the image necessary for maintaining internal coherence, thereby making less evident the contradictions and discrepancies of personal experience. In a word, auto-analysis does not bring about the elaboration of a kind of "objective self," seen from outside as being more or less reliable, insofar as it corresponds to a continuing process of readjustment and recomposition of the data, aimed primarily at stabilizing the current sense of self and possibly at articulating it further. It is thus clear that as the number and complexity of the data on hand increase, there will be an increase also in the number of contradictions and discrepancies which will become apparent in the attempt to recompose these data consistently with one's own perceived continuity and coherence. This may give us a hint as to how to understand the contrasting effects which often develop with time, on both the cognitive and emotional levels, after arriving at a consistent modification of the habitual level of awareness of the client.

At the cognitive level, the focusing on other aspects of the self, along with the reorganization of the perception of reality that this normally brings with it, reveals new critical domains of experience, making lifespan development appear as a continual "problematic shifting," in which to every increase of knowledge there corresponds the emergence of new areas of ignorance.

As far as the emotional level is concerned, the burgeoning of new levels of awareness is paralleled, almost invariably, by the growth of the sense of ambiguity in experiencing self and the world, linked in various ways to the emergence of complex emotions such as boredom, sense of the absurd, existential futility, etc. Fernando Pessoa, one of the contemporary poets who has most faithfully recorded this aspect, succeeds in providing an immediate sense of this with a phrase which many people would subscribe to if they had to explain the effect felt when faced with a "sudden" awareness of the trend of their life: "Each of us is more than one, is manifold, is a prolixity of oneself" (1982, p. 38). It is still unclear how the increase in awareness facilitates the burgeoning of such emotions, even though it seems evident that this phenomenon is in some way correlated with the diminishing of the sense of immediacy in experiencing self and the world at the very moment such experiencing, entering consciousness, becomes the object of attention.

It thus becomes evident that one must proceed with caution in bringing forward a strategy directed toward modifying habitual levels of awareness. The therapist should try to work only on those areas of experience which have shown themselves to be critical on the basis of a previous reconstruction of the basic themes of the client's personal meaning, refraining from an exaggerated intervention in other domains despite the fact that one's own conception of life might seem better and more suitable than those exhibited by the client. Moreover, within these same critical domains, one would be well advised not to proceed indiscriminately with the pursuit of awareness as such, but, quite the contrary, to be ready to grasp the minimum level of modification of viewpoint which can trigger in clients *their* own reorganization of problematic experience. It follows that all this implies on the part of the therapist the awareness of demarcation between his or her own conception of self and the evolutionary dynamics, autonomous and coherent, of the personal meaning of clients.

The therapist's awareness, on the other hand, become another problem which I should like to note in passing in concluding these reflections. In recent years, because of the progressive decline in the role of privileged, impartial observer, a whole series of studies has flourished regarding the therapist as a person (cf. Guy, 1987). One is here dealing with longitudinal studies in which, apart from the implied motivations for undertaking the career of therapist, there is the attempt to focus particularly on the effects on the person which may be brought about by the full-time practice of the profession. From the greater part of the data one may deduce that the most perturbing emotions and moods are connected, even in therapists, to an indiscriminate increase in awareness; such an increase would seem to be an integral part of psychotherapeutic work, just as being a painter involves bronchitis due to inhaling chemical vapors. We are dealing, furthermore, with an awareness derived from a rather particular dynamic. On the one hand, in fact, the therapist enters into contact with a boundless quantity of human experiences and histories which cannot be translated into other than a deeper consciousness of life and of his or her reactions when faced with it; on the other hand, however, the awareness drawn in this way is "vicarious"; that is, rather than on directly lived experience, it is based on experience derived from the life of others and as such is more susceptible of intensifying the emergence of complex and ambiguous emotions. In addition, the radical transformation of the observer–observed relationship involves the therapist even more, forcing him or her to take on a continual, and often urgent, self-referent attitude, absolutely unforeseeable until a few years ago. In this sense, the problem of the "awareness of the therapist"—of how to regulate it so that it does not reach critical levels and of how to intervene if it does—is an entirely unexplored frontier, crossing over which we find ourselves up against "the other face" of the therapeutic process. This could clarify for us many of the unsolved queries over which we ruminate concerning the "only face" that we know.

It is precisely these contrasting and unresolved aspects which, at this stage in my personal evolution as a therapist, reveal to me the interdependence between change and awareness as a critical "interface" in understanding the structure of human experience; the detailed study of such an interface could reveal to us aspects, unforeseeable today, which may lead to a level of ontological theorizing that will make that which we have sought to present in this book seem commonplace. This is what I hope will happen in the course of the next few years.

References

Abelson, R. P. (1989). Psychological status of the script concept. *American Psychologist, 36,* 715–729.

Abramson, L. Y., Seligman, M. E. P., & Teasdale, J. D. (1978). Learned helplessness in humans: Critique and reformulation. *Journal of Abnormal Psychology, 87,* 49–74.

Adams, P. L. (1973). *Obsessive children.* New York: Brunner/Mazel.

Ainsworth, M. D. S. (1985). Patterns of infant–mother attachments: Antecedents and effects on development. *Bulletin of the New York Academy of Medicine, 61,* 771–812.

Ainsworth, M. D. S., Blehar, M. C., Waters, E., & Wall, S. (1978). *Patterns of attachment.* Hillsdale, NJ: Erlbaum.

Allen, P. M. (1981). The evolutionary paradigm of dissipative structures. In E. R. Jantsch (Ed.), *Toward a unifying paradigm of physical, biological, and sociocultural evolution.* Boulder, CO: Westview.

Arciero, G. (1989). *From epistemology to ontology: A new age of cognition.* Paper presented at the American Association for the Advancement of Science, San Francisco, CA.

Arciero, G., & Mahoney, M. J. (1989). *Understanding and psychotherapy.* Unpublished manuscript, University of California, Santa Barbara.

Aries, P., & Duby, G. (1987). *Histoire de la vie privée. V. De la première guerre mondiale à nos jours.* Paris: Seuil.

Arnkoff, D. B. (1980). Psychotherapy from the perspective of cognitive theory. In M. J. Mahoney (Ed.), *Psychotherapy process.* New York: Plenum Press.

Arrindell, W. A., Emmelkamp, P. M. G., Monsma, A., & Brilman E. (1983). The role of perceived parental practices in the aetiology of phobic disorders: A controlled study. *British Journal of Psychiatry, 143,* 183–187.

Atlan, H. (1979). *Entre le cristal et la fumée.* Paris: Seuil.

Atlan, H. (1981). Hierarchical self-organization in living systems. In M. Zeleny (Ed.), *Autopoiesis: A theory of living organization.* New York: North-Holland.

Atlan, H. (1984). Disorder, complexity and meaning. In P. Livingston (Ed.), *Disorder and order.* Saratoga, CA: Anma libri.

Ballerini, A., & Rossi Monti, M. (1983). *Dopo la schizofrenia.* Milano: Feltrinelli.

Baltes, P. B. (1979). Life span developmental psychology: Some converging observations on history and theory. In P. B. Baltes & O. G. Brim (Eds.), *Life span development and behavior* (Vol. 2). New York: Academic Press.

Barkow, J. H. (1975). Prestige and culture: A biosocial interpretation. *Current Anthropology, 16,* 553–572.

Bateson, G., Jackson, D. D., Haley, J., & Weakland, J. (1956). Toward a theory of schizophrenia. *Behavioral Science, 1,* 251–264.

Baxter, L. A. (1984). Trajectories of relationship disengagement. *Journal of Social and Personal Relationships, 1,* 29–48.

Beattie-Emery, O., & Csikszentmihalyi, M. (1981). An epistemological approach to psychiatry: On the psychology/psychopathology of knowledge. *Journal of Mind and Behavior, 2,* 375–396.

Bell, S. M., & Ainsworth, M. D. S. (1972). Infant crying and maternal responsiveness. *Child Development, 43,* 1171–1190.

Berscheid, E. (1983). Emotion. In H. H. Kelley, E. Berscheid, A. Christensen, J. Harvey, T. L. Levinger, E. McClintock, A. Peplau, & D. R. Peterson, *Close relationships.* San Francisco: Freeman.

Berscheid, E., Gangestad, S. W., & Kulakowski, D. (1984). Emotion in close relationships: Implications for relationship counseling. In S. D. Brown & R. L. Lent (Eds.), *Handbook of counseling psychology.* New York: Wiley.

Bertenthal, B. I., & Fischer, K. W. (1978). Development of self-recognition in the infant. *Developmental Psychology, 14,* 44–45.

Bifulco, A. T., Brown, G. W., & Harris, T. O. (1987). Childhood loss of parent, lack of adequate parental care and adult depression: A replication. *Journal of Affective Disorders, 12,* 115–128.

Bloom, M. V. (1980). *Adolescent–parental separation.* New York: Gardner.

Bower, G. H., & Gilligan, S. G. (1979). Remembering information related to one's self. *Journal of Research in Personality, 13,* 420–432.

Bowlby, J. (1969). *Attachment and loss: Vol. 1. Attachment.* New York: Basic Books.

Bowlby, J. (1973). *Attachment and loss: Vol. 2. Separation: Anxiety and anger.* New York: Basic Books.

Bowlby, J. (1977). The making and breaking of affectional bonds: I. Etiology and psychopathology in the light of attachment theory. *British Journal of Psychiatry, 130,* 201–210.

Bowlby, J. (1980). *Attachment and loss: Vol. 3. Loss, sadness and depression.* London: Hogarth Press.

Bowlby, J. (1983). *Attachment and loss: Vol. 1. Attachment* (2nd ed.). London: Hogarth Press.

Bowlby, J. (1985). The role of childhood experience in cognitive disturbance. In M. J. Mahoney & A. Freeman (Eds.), *Cognition and psychotherapy.* New York: Plenum Press.

Bowlby, J. (1988). Developmental psychiatry comes of age. In *A secure base.* New York: Basic Books.

Braudel, F. (1979). *Civilisation matérielle, économie et capitalisme (XV–XVIII siècle). Les structures du quotidien: Le possible et l'impossible.* Paris: Armand Colin.

Brazelton, T. B. (1983). Precursors for the development of emotions in early infancy. In R. Plutchik & A. Kellerman (Eds.), *Emotion: Theory, research and experience* (Vol. 2). New York: Academic Press.

Brazelton, T. B., Koslowaki, B., & Main, M. (1974). The origins of reciprocity: The early mother–infant interaction. In M. Lewis & L. A. Rosenblum (Eds.), *The effect of the infant on its caregivers.* New York: Wiley.

Brent, S. B. (1978). Prigogine's model for self-organization in nonequilibrium systems: Its relevance for developmental psychology. *Human Development, 21,* 374–387.

Brent, S. B. (1984). *Psychological and social structures.* Hillsdale, NJ: Erlbaum.

Bretherton, I. (1984). *Symbolic play: The development of social understanding.* New York: Academic Press.

Bretherton, I. (1985). Attachment theory: Retrospect and prospect. In I. Bretherton & E. Waters (Eds.), *Growing points of attachment theory and research* (Monographs of the Society for Research in Child Development, Serial No. 209, Vol. 50, Nos. 1–2). Chicago: University of Chicago Press.

Bretherton, I., & Waters, E. (Eds.). (1985). *Growing points of attachment theory and research* (Monographs of the Society for Research in Child Development, Serial No. 209, Vol. 50, Nos. 1–2). Chicago: University of Chicago Press.

Broughton, J. (1980). Development of concepts of self, mind, reality and knowledge. *New Directions for Child Development, 24,* 75–100.

Brown, G. W. (1982). Early loss and depression. In C. M. Parkes & J. Stevenson-Hinde (Eds.), *The place of attachment in human behavior.* London: Tavistock.

Buck, R. (1984). *The communication of emotion.* New York: Guilford Press.

Bugental, J. F. T., & Bugental, E. (1984). A fate worse than death: The fear of changing. *Psychotherapy, 21,* 543–549.

Buss, A. H. (1987). Personality: Primate heritage and human distinctiveness. In J. Aronoff, A. I. Rabin, & R. A. Zucker (Eds.), *The emergence of personality.* New York: Springer.

Buss, A. H. (1988). *Personality: Evolutionary heritage and human distinctiveness.* Hillsdale, NJ: Erlbaum.

Campbell, D. T. (1974). Evolutionary epistemology. In P. A. Schilpp (Ed.), *The philosophy of Karl Popper.* La Salle, IL: Library of Living Philosophers.

Campos, J., & Stenberg, C. (1981). Perception, appraisal, and emotion: The onset of social referencing. In M. Lamb & L. Sherrod (Eds.), *Infant social cognition.* Hillsdale, NJ: Erlbaum.

Campos, J. J., & Caplovitz Barrett, K. (1984). Toward a new understanding of emotions and their development. In C. E. Izard, J. Kagan, & R. B. Zajonc (Eds.), *Emotions, cognition, and behavior.* Cambridge: Cambridge University Press.

Carlson, L., & Carlson, R. (1984). Affect and psychological magnification: Derivations from Tomkins' script theory. *Journal of Personality, 52,* 36–45.

Carlson, R. (1981). Studies in script theory: I. Adult analogs of a childhood nuclear scene. *Journal of Personality and Social Psychology, 40,* 501–510.

Cassidy, J., & Kobak, R. R. (1988). Avoidance and its relation to other defensive processes. In J. Belsky & T. Nezworski (Eds.), *Clinical implications of attachments.* Hillsdale, NJ: Erlbaum.

Ceruti, M. (1989). *La danza che crea: Evoluzione e cognizione nell'epistemologia genetica.* Milano: Feltrinelli.

Chatoor, I. (1989). Infantile anorexia nervosa: A developmental disorder of separation and individuation. *Journal of the American Academy of Psychoanalysis, 17,* 43–64.

Chatoor, I., Egan, J., Getson, P., Menvielle, E., & O'Donnell, R. (1988). Mother–infant interactions in infantile anorexia nervosa. *Journal of the American Academy of Child and Adolescent Psychiatry, 27,* 535–540.

Cicchetti, D., & Pogge-Hesse, P. (1981). The relation between emotion and cognitions in infant development: Past, present, and future perspectives. In M. Lamb & L. Sherrod (Eds.), *Infant social cognition: Empirical and theoretical considerations.* Hillsdale, NJ: Erlbaum

Cioran, E. M. (1981). *Ecartèlement* (quotations from Italian translation *Squartamento*). Milano: Adelphi.

Claiborn, C. D. (1982). Interpretation and change in counseling. *Journal of Counseling Psychology, 29,* 439–453.

Claiborn, C. D., & Dowd, T. E. (1985). Attributional interpretations in counseling: Content versus discrepancy. *Journal of Counseling Psychology, 32,* 188–196.

Clark, D. A., & Bolton, D. (1985). Obsessive-compulsive adolescents and their parents: A psychometric study. *Journal of Child Psychology, Psychiatry and Allied Disciplines, 26,* 267–276.

Clark, M. S., & Reis, H. T. (1988). Interpersonal processes in close relationships. *Annual Review of Psychology, 39,* 609–672.

Collins, A. M., & Loftus, E. F. (1975). A spreading activation theory of semantic processing. *Psychological Review, 82,* 407–428.

Cooley, C. H. (1902). *Human nature and the social order.* New York: Scribner.

Cowan, N. (1988). Evolving conceptions of memory storage, selective attention, and their mutual coustraints within the human information-processing system. *Psychological Bulletin, 104,* 163–191.

Csikszentmihalyi, M., & Figurski, T. J. (1982). Self-awareness and aversive experience in every day life. *Journal of Personality, 50,* 15–28.

Damon, W., & Hart, D. (1982). The development of self-understanding from infancy through adolescence. *Child Development, 53,* 841–864.

Davis, M. D. (1983). *Game theory.* New York: Basic Books.

Dell, P. F., & Goolishian, H. A. (1981). "Order through fluctuation": An evolutionary epistemology for human systems. *Australian Journal of Family Therapy, 2,* 175–184.

Dennett, D. (1978). *Brainstorms.* Montgomery, VT: Bradford Books.

Dixon, N. (1981). *Preconscious processing.* New York: Wiley.

Dobert, R., Habermas, J., & Nunner-Winkler, G. (1987). The development of the self. In J. M. Broughton (Ed.), *Critical theories of psychological development.* New York: Plenum Press.

Draguns, J. G. (1984). Microgenesis by any other name. . . . In W. D. Froehlich, G. Smith, J. G. Draguns, & U. Hentschel (Eds.), *Psychological processes in cognition and personality.* Washington: Hemisphere.

Duck, S. W. (1982). A topography of relationship disengagement and dissolution. In S. W. Duck (Ed.), *Personal relationships 4: Dissolving personal relationships.* New York: Academic Press.

Eigen, M., & Winkler, R. (1981). *Laws of the game.* New York: Harper & Row.

Ekman, P. (1972). Universal and cultural differences in facial expression of emotion. In J. K. Cole (Ed.), *Nebraska symposium on motivation* (Vol. 19). Lincoln: University of Nebraska Press.

Ekman, P. (1984). Expression and the nature of emotion. In K. R. Scherer & P. Ekman (Eds.), *Approaches to emotion.* Hillsdale, NJ: Erlbaum.

Ekman, P., Levenson, R. W., & Friesen, N. V. (1983). Autonomic nervous system activity distinguishes among emotions. *Science, 221,* 1208–1210.

Emde, R. N. (1984). Levels of meaning for infant emotions: A biosocial view. In K. R. Scherer & P. Ekman (Eds.), *Approaches to emotion.* Hillsdale, NJ: Erlbaum.

Faust, D., & Miner, R. A. (1986). The empiricist and his new clothes: DSM-III in perspective. *American Journal of Psychiatry, 143,* 962–967.

Faust, D., & Ziskin, J. (1988). The expert witness in psychology and psychiatry. *Science, 241,* 31–35.

Field, T. (1985). Attachment as psychobiological attunement: Being on the same wavelength. In M. Reite & T. Field (Eds.), *The psychobiology of attachment and separation.* New York: Academic Press.

Field, T., & Reite, M. (1985). The psychobiology of attachment and separation: A summary. In M. Reite & T. Field (Eds.), *The psychobiology of attachment and separation.* New York: Academic Press.

Field, T. M., Woodson, R., Greenberg, R., & Cohen, D. (1982). Discrimination and imitation of facial expressions by neonates. *Science, 218,* 179–181.

Forsyth, D. R., & Strong, S. R. (1986). The scientific study of counseling and psychotherapy: A unificationist view. *American Psychologist, 41,* 113–119.

Fox, N. A., & Davidson, R. J. (Eds.) (1984). *The psychobiology of affective development.* Hillsdale, NJ: Erlbaum.

Gadamer, H. G. (1976). *Philosophical hermeneutics.* Berkeley: University of California Press.

Gadamer, H. G. (1979). *Truth and method.* London: Sheed & Ward.

Gallup, G. G. (1970). Chimpanzees: Self-recognition. *Science, 167,* 86–87.

Gallup, G. G. (1977). Self-recognition in primates. *American Psychologist, 32,* 329–338.

Gallup, G. G., McClure, M. K., Hill, S. D., & Bundt, R. A. (1971). Capacity for self-recognition in differentially reared chimpanzees. *Psychological Record, 21,* 69–74.

Gallup, G. G., & Suarez, S. (1986). Self-awareness and the emergence of mind in humans and other primates. In J. Suls & A. G. Greenwald (Eds.), *Psychological perspectives on the self* (Vol. 3). Hillsdale, NJ: Erlbaum.

Gardner, B. T. & Gardner, R. A. (1971). Two-way communication with an infant chimpanzee. In A. M. Schrier & F. Stollnitz (Eds.), *Behavior of nonhuman primates: Modern research trends* (Vol. 4). New York: Academic Press.

Giele, J. Z. (1980). Adulthood as transcendence of age and sex. In N. J. Smelser & E. H. Erikson (Eds.), *Themes of work and love in adulthood.* Cambridge, MA: Harvard University Press.

Gilligan, S. G., & Bower, G. H. (1984). Cognitive consequences of emotional arousal. In C. E. Izard, J. Kagan, & R. B. Zajonc (Eds.),

Emotions, cognition and behavior. Cambridge: Cambridge University Press.

Glasser, R. (1982). Instructional psychology. *American Psychologist, 37,* 292–305.

Gould, R. L. (1978). *Transformations: Growth and change in adult life.* New York: Simon & Schuster.

Gould, S. J. (1980). *The panda's thumb: More reflections in natural history.* New York: Norton.

Greenberg, L. S. (1984). A task analysis of intrapersonal conflict resolution. In L. N. Rice & L. S. Greenberg (Eds.), *Patterns of change: Intensive analysis of psychotherapy process.* New York: Guilford Press.

Greenberg, L. S., & Safran, J. D. (1987). *Emotion in psychotherapy.* New York: Guilford Press.

Guidano, V. F. (1988). A systems, process-oriented approach to cognitive therapy. In K. S. Dobson (Ed.), *Handbook of cognitive-behavioral therapies.* New York: Guilford Press.

Guidano, V. F. (1987). *Complexity of the self.* New York: Guilford Press.

Guidano, V. F. (1991). Affective change events in a cognitive therapy system approach. In J. D. Safran & L. S. Greenberg (Eds.), *Emotion, psychotherapy, and change.* New York: Guilford Press.

Guidano, V. F., & Liotti, G. (1983). *Cognitive processes and emotional disorders.* New York: Guilford Press.

Guidano, V. F., & Liotti, G. (1985). A constructivistic foundation for cognitive therapy. In M. J. Mahoney & A. Freeman (Eds.), *Cognition and psychotherapy.* New York: Plenum.

Guy, J. D. (1987). *The personal life of the psychotherapist.* New York: Wiley.

Habermas, J. (1979). *Communication and the evolution of society.* London: Heinemann.

Habermas, J. (1981). *Theorie des kommunikativen handelns I–II.* Frankfurt am Main: Suhrkamp.

Hafner, R. J. (1986). *Marriage and mental illness.* New York: Guilford Press.

Hamlyn, D. (1974). Person perception and our understanding of others. In T. Mischel (Ed.), *Understanding other persons.* Totowa, NJ: Rowman & Littlefield.

Harter, S. (1983). Development perspectives on the self-system. In E. M. Hetherington (Ed.), *Handbook of child psychology: Vol. 4. Socialization, personality and social development.* New York: Wiley.

Harvey, J. H., Flanary, R., & Morgan, M. (1986). Vivid memories of vivid loves gone by. *Journal of Social and Personal Relationships, 3,* 359–373.

Hasher, L., & Zacks, R. T. (1979). Automatic and effortful processes in memory. *Journal of Experimental Psychology: General, 108,* 356–388.

Hasher, L., & Zacks, R. T. (1984). Automatic processing of fundamental information. *American Psychologist, 39,* 1372–1388.

Haviland, J. M. (1984). Thinking and feeling in Woolf's writing: From childhood to adulthood. In C. E. Izard, J. Kagan, & R. B. Zajonc (Eds.), *Emotions, cognition and behavior.* Cambridge: Cambridge University Press.

Hayek, F. A. (1952). *The sensory order.* Chicago: University of Chicago Press.

Hayek, F. A. (1978). *New studies in philosophy, politics, economics and the history of ideas.* Chicago: University of Chicago Press.

Hazan, C., & Shaver, P. (1987). Romantic love conceptualized as an attachment process. *Journal of Personality and Social Psychology, 52,* 511–524.

Henderson, S. (1982). The significance of social relationships in the etiology of neurosis. In C. M. Parker & J. Stevenson-Hinde (Eds.), *The place of attachment in human behavior.* London: Tavistock.

Henderson, S., Byrbe, D. G., & Duncan-Jones, P. (1981). *Neurosis and the social environment.* New York: Academic Press.

Hinde, R. A. (1979). *Towards understanding relationships.* London: Academic Press.

Hofer, M. A. (1984). Relationships as regulators: A psychobiologic perspective on bereavement. *Psychosomatic Medicine, 46,* 183–197.

Hoffman, M. L. (1975). Development synthesis of affect and cognition and its implications for alternistic motivation. *Developmental Psychology, 11,* 607–622.

Hoffman, M. L. (1978). Toward a theory of empathic arousal and development. In M. Lewis & L. A. Rosenblum (Eds.), *The development of affect.* New York: Plenum Press.

Hoffman, M. L. (1984). Interaction of affect and cognition in empathy. In C. E. Izard, J. Kagan, & R. B. Zajonc (Eds.), *Emotions, cognition and behavior.* Cambridge: Cambridge University Press.

House, J. S., Landis, K. R., & Umberson, D. (1988). Social relationships and health. *Science, 241,* 540–545.

Ianniruberto, A., & Tajani, E. (1981). Ultrasonographic study of fetal movements. In *Seminars in perinatology.* New York: Grune & Stratton.

Izard, C. E. (1977). *Human emotions.* New York: Plenum Press.

Izard, C. E. (1980). The emergence of emotions and the development of consciousness in infancy. In J. M. Davidson & R. J. Davidson (Eds.), *The psychobiology of consciousness.* New York: Plenum Press.

Izard, C. E., & Buechler, S. (1980). Aspects of consciousness and personality in terms of differential emotions theory. In R. Plutchik & H. Kellerman (Eds.), *Emotion: Theory, research and experience: Vol. 1. Theories of emotion.* New York: Academic Press.

Izard, C. E., & Schwartz, G. M. (1986). Patterns of emotion in depression. In M. Rutter, C. E. Izard, & P. B. Read (Eds.), *Depression in young people.* New York: Guilford Press.

James, W. (1980). The consciousness of self. In *Principles of psychology* (Vol. 1). New York: Holt, Rinehart & Winston.

Jantsch, E. (1980). *The self-organizing universe.* New York: Pergamon Press.

Johnson, F. (1985). The western concept of self. In A. J. Marsella, G. DeVos, & F. L. K. Hsu, *Culture and self.* London: Tavistock.

Johnson, M. (1987). *The body in the mind: The bodily basis of meaning, imagination and reason.* Chicago: University of Chicago Press.

Kegan, R. (1982). *The evolving self.* Cambridge, MA: Harvard University Press.

Kelley, H. H., Berscheid, E., Christensen, A., Harvey, J., Huston, T. L., Levinger, G., McClintock, E., Peplau, A., & Peterson, D. R. (1983). *Close relationships.* San Francisco: Freeman.

Ketterer, M. W. (1985). Awareness: I. The natural ecology of subjective experience and the mind–brain problem revisited. *Journal of Mind and Behavior, 6,* 469–514.

Klinnert, M., Campos, J., Sorce, J., Emde, R., & Svejda, M. (1983). Emotions as behavior regulators: Social referencing in infancy. In R. Plutchik & H. Kellerman (Eds.), *Emotion: Theory, research and experience: Vol. 2. Emotions in early development.* New York: Academic Press.

Kummer, H. (1979). On the value of social relationships to nonhuman primates: A heuristic scheme. In M. Von Cranach, K. Foppa, W. Lepenies, & D. Ploog (Eds.), *Human ethology.* Cambridge: Cambridge University Press.

La Rochefoucauld, F. de. (1959). *Maxims.* London: Penguin. (Original work published 1678)

Lakatos, I. (1974). Falsification and the methodology of scientific research programmes. In I. Lakatos & A. Musgrave (Eds.), *Criticism and the growth of knowledge.* Cambridge: Cambridge University Press.

Lakoff, G. (1987). *Women, fire, and dangerous things: What categories reveal about the mind.* Chicago: University of Chicago Press.

Lakoff, G., & Johnson, M. (1980). *Metaphors we live by.* Chicago: University of Chicago Press.

Lambert, M. J. (1989). The individual therapist's contribution to psychotherapy process and outcome. *Clinical Psychology Review, 9,* 469–485.

Lane, R. D., & Schwartz, G. E. (1987). Levels of emotional awareness: A cognitive-development theory and its application to psychopathology. *American Journal of Psychiatry, 144,* 133–143.

Lang, P. J. (1984). Cognition in emotion: Concept and action. In C. E.

Izard, J. Kagan, & R. B. Zajonc (Eds.), *Emotions, cognitions and behavior.* Cambridge: Cambridge University Press.

Lee, L. (1984). Sequences in separation: A framework for investigating endings of personal (romantic) relationships. *Journal of Social and Personal Relationships, 1,* 49–73.

Lerner, R. M. (1984). *On the nature of human plasticity.* Cambridge: Cambridge University Press.

Lerner, R. M., & Busch-Rossnagel, N. A. (Eds.). (1981). *Individuals as producers of their development: A life-span perspective.* New York: Academic Press.

Levenson, R. W., & Gottman, J. M. (1983). Marital interaction: Physiological linkage and affective exchange. *Journal of Personality and Social Psychology, 45,* 587–597.

Levine, M. (1942). *Psychotherapy in medical practice.* New York: Macmillan.

Levinson, D. J. (1978). *The seasons of a man's life.* New York: Knopf.

Levinson, D. J. (1986). A conception of adult development. *American Psychologist, 41,* 3–13.

Lewis, H. B. (1986). The role of shame in depression. In M. Rutter, C. E. Izard, & P. B. Read (Eds.), *Depression in young people.* New York: Guilford Press.

Lewis, H. B. (1988). The role of shame in symptom formation. In M. Clynes & J. Panksepp (Eds.), *Emotions and psychopathology.* New York: Plenum Press.

Lewis, M., & Brooks-Gunn, J. (1979). *Social cognition and the acquisition of self.* New York: Plenum Press.

Linville, P. W. (1985). Self-complexity and affective extremity: Don't put all of your eggs in one cognitive basket. *Social Cognition, 3,* 94–120.

Linville, P. W. (1987). Self-complexity as a cognitive buffer against stress-related illness and depression. *Journal of Personality and Social Psychology, 52,* 663–676.

Lorenz, K. (1973). *Die ruckseite des spiegels.* Munich: Piper. (English translation: *Behind the mirror.* New York: Harcourt Brace Jovanovich, 1977)

Lutkenhaus, P., Grossmann, K. E., & Grossmann, K. (1985). Infant–mother attachment at 12 months and style of interaction with a stranger at the age of three years. *Child Development, 56,* 1538–1572.

Mahoney, M. J. (1980). Psychotherapy and the structure of personal revolutions. In M. J. Mahoney (Ed.), *Psychotherapy process.* New York: Plenum Press.

Mahoney, M. J. (1981). Clinical psychology and scientific inquiry. *International Journal of Psychology, 16,* 257–274.

Mahoney, M. J. (1984). Psychoanalysis and behaviorism: The yin and yang of determinism. In H. Arkowitz & S. Messer (Eds.), *Psychoanalytic and behavior therapy: Is integration possible?* New York: Plenum Press.

Mahoney, M. J. (1985). Psychotherapy and human change processes. In M. J. Mahoney & A. Freeman (Eds.), *Cognition and psychotherapy*. New York: Plenum Press.

Mahoney, M. J. (1988). Constructive metatheory: I. Basic features and historical foundations. *International Journal of Personal Construct Psychology, 1*, 1–35.

Mahoney, M. J. (1991). *Human change processes: The scientific foundations of psychotherapy*. New York: Basic Books.

Mahoney, M. J., & Gabriel, T. J. (1987). Psychotherapy and cognitive sciences: An evolving alliance. *Journal of Cognitive Psychotherapy, 1*, 39–59.

Mahoney, M. J., & Lyddon, W. L. (1988). Recent developments in cognitive approaches to counseling and psychotherapy. *Counseling Psychologist, 16*, 190–234.

Mahoney, M. J., Lyddon, W. J., & Alford, D. J. (1989). An evaluation of the rational-emotive theory of psychotherapy. In M. E. Bernard & R. DiGiuseppe (Eds.), *Inside rational-emotive therapy*. New York: Academic Press.

Mahoney, M. J., Miller, M. & Arciero, G. (in press). Constructive metatheory and the nature of mental representation. *Journal of Mental Imagery*.

Main, M., Kaplan, N., & Cassidy, J. (1985). Security in infancy, childhood, and adulthood: A move to the level of representation. In I. Bretherton & E. Waters (Eds.), *Growing points of attachment theory and research* (Monographs of the Society for Research in Child Development, Serial No. 209, Vol. 50, Nos. 1–2). Chicago: University of Chicago Press.

Main, M., & Weston, D. R. (1982). Avoidance of the attachment figure in infancy: Descriptions and interpretations. In C. M. Parkes & J. Stevenson-Hinde (Eds.), *The place of attachment in human behavior*. London: Tavistock.

Makhlouf-Norris, F. & Norris, H. (1972). The obsessive-compulsive syndrome as a neurotic device for the reduction of self-uncertainty. *British Journal of Psychiatry, 121*, 277–288.

Malatesta, C. Z., & Clayton Culver, L. (1984). Thematic and affective content in the lives of adult women: Patterns of change and continuity. In C. Z. Malatesta & C. E. Izard (Eds.), *Emotion in adult development*. Beverly Hills, CA: Sage.

Mancuso, J. C., & Ceely, S. G. (1980). The self as memory processing. *Cognitive Therapy and Research, 4*, 1–25.

Markus, H. (1977). Self-schemata and processing information about the self. *Journal of Personality and Social Psychology, 35*, 63–78.

Markus, H., & Nurius, P. (1986). Possible selves. *American Psychologist, 41,* 954–969.

Marmor, J. (1983). Systems thinking in psychiatry: Some theoretical and clinical implications. *American Journal of Psychiatry, 140,* 833–838.

Marris, P. (1982). Attachment and society. In C. M. Parkes & J. Stevenson-Hinde (Eds.), *The place of attachment in human behavior.* London: Tavistock.

Marshall, G. D., & Zimbardo, P. G. (1979). Affective consequences of inadequately explained physiological arousal. *Journal of Personality and Social Psychology, 6,* 970–988.

Maslach, C. (1979). Negative emotional biasing of unexplained arousal. *Journal of Personality and Social Psychology, 6,* 953–969.

Maturana, H. (1978). Biology of language: The epistemology of reality. In G. A. Miller & E. Lenneberg (Eds.), *Psychology and biology of language and thought: Essays in honor of Eric Lenneberg.* New York: Academic Press.

Maturana, H. (1986). *Ontology of observing: The biological foundations of self-consciousness and the physical domain of existence.* Unpublished manuscript, University of Chile, Santiago.

Maturana, H. (1988a). Reality: The search for objectivity, or the quest for a compelling argument. *Irish Journal of Psychology, 9,* 25–82.

Maturana, H. (1988b). Ontologia del conversar. *Terapía Psicológica, 10,* 15–23.

Maturana, H., & Varela, F. (1980). *Autopoiesis and cognition: The realization of living.* Dordrecht: Reidel.

Maturana, H., & Varela, F. (1987). *The tree of knowledge.* Boston: Shambhala.

McGuire, M. T., & Troisi, A. (1987). Psychological regulation–deregulation and psychiatric disorders. *Ethology and Sociobiology, 8,* 9s–25s.

Mead, G. H. (1934). *Mind, self and society.* Chicago: University of Chicago Press.

Melnechuck, T (1988). Emotions, brain, immunity, and health: A review. In M. Clynes & J. Panksepp (Eds.), *Emotions and psychopathology.* New York: Plenum Press.

Meltzoff, A. N., & Borton, R. W. (1979). Intermodal matching by human neonates. *Nature, 282,* 403–404.

Meltzoff, A. N., & Moore, M. K. (1985). Cognitive foundations and social functions of imitation and intermodal representation in infancy. In J. Mehler & R. Fox (Eds.), *Neonate cognition.* Hillsdale, NJ: Erlbaum.

Miall, D. S. (1986). Emotions and the self: The context of remembering. *British Journal of Psychology, 77,* 389–397.

Milani Comparetti, A. (1981). The neurophysiologic and clinical implications of studies on fetal mother behavior. In *Seminars in perinatology.* New York: Grune & Stratton.

Miller, G. A. (1981). Trends and debates in cognitive psychology. *Cognition,* 10, 215–225.

Mineka, S., Suomi, S. J., & De Lizio, R. (1981). Multiple separations in adolescent monkeys: An opponent-process interpretation. *Journal of Experimental Psychology,* 110, 56–85.

Minuchin, S. (1974). *Families and family therapy.* Cambridge, MA: Harvard University Press.

Minuchin, S., Rosman, B. L., & Baker, L. (1978). *Psychosomatic families: Anorexia nervosa in context.* Cambridge, MA: Harvard University Press.

Morin, E. (1986). *La méthode: III. La connaissance de la connaissance.* Paris: Seuil.

Morin, E., & Piattelli Palmarini, M. (1974). *L'unité de l'homme.* Paris: Seuil.

Nagel, T. (1979). *Mortal questions.* Cambridge: Cambridge University Press.

Nelson, K., & Ross, G. (1982). The generalities and specifics of long-term memory in infants and young children. In M. Perlmutter (Ed.), *Naturalistic approaches to memory.* San Francisco: Jossey-Bass.

Nicolis, G., & Prigogine, I. (1977). *Self-organization in nonequilibrium systems: From dissipative structures to order through fluctuations.* New York: Wiley.

Nisbett, R. E., & Wilson, T. D. (1977). Telling more than we can know: Verbal reports on mental processes. *Psychological Review,* 84, 231–259.

Olafson, A. F. (1988). *Heidegger and the philosophy of mind.* New Haven, CT: Yale University Press.

Panksepp, J. (1988). Brain emotional circuits and psychopathologies. In M. Clynes & J. Panksepp (Eds.), *Emotions and psychopathology.* New York: Plenum Press.

Panksepp, J., Siviy, S., & Normansell, L. A. (1985). Brain opioids and social emotions. In M. Reite & T. Field (Eds.), *The psychobiology of attachment and separation.* New York: Academic Press.

Parker, G. (1979). Reported parental characteristics of agoraphobics and social phobics. *British Journal of Psychiatry,* 135, 555–560.

Parker, G. (1983a). Parental "affectionless control" as an antecedent to adult depression. *Archives of General Psychiatry,* 50, 956–960.

Parker, G. (1983b). *Parental overprotection: A risk factor in psychosocial development.* London: Grune & Stratton.

Parkes, C. M. (1972). *Bereavement: Studies of grief in adult life.* London: Tavistock.

Parkes, C. M. (1982). Attachment and the prevention of mental disorders.

In C. M. Parkes & I. Stevenson-Hinde (Eds.), *The place of attachment in human behavior*. London: Tavistock.

Parkes, C. M., & Weiss, R. S. (1983). *Recovery from bereavement*. New York: Basic Books.

Passingham, R. (1982). *The human primate*. San Francisco: Freeman.

Pessoa, F. (1987). *Il libro dell'inquietudine*. Milano: Feltrinelli.

Piaget, J. (1971). *Biology and knowledge*. Chicago: University of Chicago Press.

Pirandello, L. (1987). *The late Mattia Pascal*. New York: Dedalus. (Original work published 1904)

Plutchik, R. (1984). Emotions: A general psychoevolutionary theory. In K. R. Scherer & P. Ekman (Eds.), *Approaches to emotions*. Hillsdale, NJ: Erlbaum.

Popper, K. R. (1972). *Objective knowledge: An evolutionary approach*. Oxford: Clarendon Press. (Rev. ed., 1979)

Popper, K. R. (1975). The rationality of scientific revolutions. In R. Harré (Ed.), *Problems of scientific revolutions*. Oxford: Clarendon Press.

Popper, K. R. (1982). The place of mind in nature. In R. Q. Elvee (Ed.), *Mind in nature*. San Francisco: Harper & Row.

Popper, K. R., & Eccles, J. C. (1977). *The self and its brain*. New York: Springer.

Posner, M. I., & Snyder, C. R. R. (1975). Facilitation and inhibition in the processing of signals. In P. M. A. Rabbit & S. Dornic (Eds.), *Attention and performance* (Vol. 5). New York: Academic Press.

Prigogine, I. (1973). Irreversibility as a symmetry-breaking process. *Nature, 246*, 67–71.

Prigogine, I. (1976). Order through fluctuations. Self-organization and social systems. In E. Jantsch & C. H Waddington (Eds.), *Evolution and consciousness: Human systems in transition*. Reading, MA: Addison-Wesley.

Putnam, H. (1981). *Reason, truth and history*. Cambridge: Cambridge University Press.

Radnitzky, G., & Bartley, W. W. III (Eds.). (1987). *Evolutionary epistemology, theory of rationality, and the sociology of knowledge*. La Salle, IL: Open Court.

Raphael, B. (1983). *The anatomy of bereavement*. New York: Basic Books.

Reda, M. A. (1984). Cognitive organization and antidepressants. In M. A. Reda & M. J. Mahoney (Eds.), *Cognitive psychotherapies: Recent developments*. Cambridge, MA: Ballinger.

Reda, M. A. (1986). *Sistemi cognitivi complessi e psicoterapia*. Roma: La Nuova Italia Scientifica.

Reda, M. A., Arciero, G., & Blanco, S. (1986). Organizzazioni cognitive, strutture psicofisiologiche e diagnosi di schizofrenia. *Rivista di Psichiatria, 21*, 142–158.

Reda, M. A., Blanco, S., Guidano, V. F., & Mahoney, M. J. (1988, November). *Physiological deregulation and psychological disorders: Data from the clinical use of mirror time.* Paper presented at the 22nd Annual Convention of the Association for Advancement of Behavior Therapy, New York, NY.

Reed, G. F. (1969). "Under-inclusion": A characteristic of obsessional personality disorder: I–II. *British Journal of Psychiatry, 115,* 781–790.

Reed, G. F. (1985). *Obsessional experience and compulsive behavior. A cognitive-structural approach.* New York: Academic Press.

Reite, M., & Field, T. (Eds.). (1985). *The psychobiology of attachment and separation.* New York: Academic Press.

Reynolds, P. C. (1981). *On the evolution of human behavior.* Los Angeles: University of California Press.

Ritter, W. (1979). Cognition and the brain. In H. Begleiter (Ed.), *Evoked brain potentials and behavior.* New York: Plenum Press.

Rosenberg, S., & Gara, M. (1985). The multiplicity of personal identity. In P. Shaver (Ed.), *Review of personality and social psychology* (Vol. 6). Beverly Hills, CA: Sage.

Rosenblum, L. A., & Paully, G. S. (1987). Primate models of separation-induced depression. *Psychiatric Clinics of North America, 10,* 437–447.

Safran, J. D., & Greenberg, L. S. (Eds.). (1991). *Emotion, psychotherapy, and change.* New York: Guilford Press.

Saint-Exupéry, A. de. (1979). *The wisdom of the sands.* Chicago: University of Chicago Press. (Original work published 1942)

Salzman, L. (1973). *The obsessive personality.* New York: Aronson.

Sander, L. W. (1975). Infant and caretaking environment. In E. J. Anthony (Ed.), *Explorations in child psychiatry.* New York: Plenum Press.

Schrag, C. O. (1986). *Communicative praxis and the space of subjectivity.* Indianapolis: Indiana University Press.

Schwartz, G. E. (1987). Personality and the unification of psychology and modern physics: A systems approach. In J. Aronoff, A. I. Rabin, & R. A. Zucker (Eds.), *The emergence of personality.* New York: Springer.

Schwartz, R. M., & Trabasso, T. (1984). Children's understanding of emotions. In C. E. Izard, J. Kagan, & R. B. Zajonc (Eds.), *Emotions, cognition and behavior.* Cambridge: Cambridge University Press.

Seligman, M. E. P., & Peterson, C. (1986). A learned helplessness perspective on childhood depression: Theory and research. In M. Rutter, C. E. Izard, & P. B. Read (Eds.), *Depression in young people.* New York: Guilford Press.

Selman, R. (1980). *The growth of interpersonal understanding.* New York: Academic Press.

Shanon, B. (1987). On the place of representations in cognition. In D. N.

Perkins, J. Lochhead, & J. Bishop (Eds.), *Thinking: The second international conference.* Hillsdale, NJ: Erlbaum.

Shanon, B. (1988). Semantic representation of meaning: A critique. *Psychological Bulletin, 104,* 70–83.

Shaver, P., Hazan, C., & Bradshaw, D. (1988). Love as attachment. In R. J. Stenberg & M. L. Barnes (Eds.), *The psychology of love.* New Haven, CT: Yale University Press.

Sheehy, G. (1976). *Passages: Predictable crises of adult life.* New York: Bantam Books.

Sluzki, C. E., & Veron, E. (1976). The double bind as a universal pathogenic situation. In C. E. Sluzki & D. C. Ransom (Eds.), *Double bind.* New York: Grune & Stratton.

Small, S. A., & Robins, C. J. (1988). The influence of induced depressed mood on visual recognition thresholds: Predictive ambiguity of associative network models of mood and cognition. *Cognitive Therapy and Research, 12,* 295–304.

Smelser, N. J. (1980). Vicissitudes of work and love in Anglo-American society. In N. J. Smelser & E. H. Erikson (Eds.), *Themes of work and love in adulthood.* Cambridge, MA: Harvard University Press.

Smith, M. B. (1985). The metaphorical basis of selfhood. In A. J. Marsella, G. DeVos, & F. L. K. Hsu, *Culture and self.* London: Tavistock.

Smith, M. B. (1978a). What it means to be human. In R. Fitzgerald (Ed.), *What it means to be human.* Rushcutters' Bay, NSW, Australia: Pergamon Press.

Smith, M. B. (1978b). Perspectives on selfhood. *American Psychologist, 33,* 1053–1063.

Solomon, R. L. (1980). The opponent-process theory of acquired motivation. *American Psychologist, 35,* 691–712.

Sommer, R. (1982). The district attorney's dilemma: Experimental games and real world of plea bargaining. *American Psychologist, 37,* 526–532.

Spitzer, H., Desimone, R., & Moran, J. (1988). Increased attention enhances both behavioral and neuronal performance. *Science, 240,* 338–340.

Sroufe, L. A., & Rutter, M. (1984). The domain of developmental psychopathology. *Child Development, 55,* 17–29.

Stayton, D. J., Hogan, R., & Ainsworth, M. D. S. (1971). Infant obedience and maternal behavior: The origins of socialization reconsidered. *Child Development, 42,* 1057–1069.

Stenberg, R. J., & Barnes, M. L. (1985). Real and ideal others in romantic relationships: Is four a crowd? *Journal of Personality and Social Psychology, 49,* 1586–1608.

Stewart, A. J., & Healy, J. M. (1984). Processing affective responses to life experiences: The development of the adult self. In C. Z. Malatesta &

C. E. Izard (Eds.), *Emotion in adult development*. Beverly Hills, CA: Sage.

Stone, G. L. (1984). Reaction: In defense of the artificial. *Journal of Counseling Psychology, 31,* 108–110.

Suomi, S. G. (1984). The development of affect in rhesus monkeys. In N. A. Fox & R. J. Davidson, *The psychobiology of affective development*. Hillsdale, NJ: Erlbaum.

Swidler, A. (1980). Love and adulthood in American culture. In N. J. Smelser & E. H. Erikson (Eds.), *Themes of work and love in adulthood*. Cambridge, MA: Harvard University Press.

Tesser, A. (1987). Toward a self-evaluation maintenance model of social behavior. In L. Berkowitz (Ed.), *Advances in experimental social psychology* (Vol. 20). New York: Academic Press.

Tomkins, S. S. (1978). Script theory: Differential magnification of affects. In H. E. Howe & M. M. Page (Eds.), *Nebraska symposium on motivation* (Vol. 24). Lincoln: University of Nebraska Press.

Tomkins, S. S. (1987). Script theory. In J. Aronoff, A. I. Rabin, & R. A. Zucker (Eds.), *The emergence of personality*. New York: Springer.

Trevarthen, C. (1979). Instincts for human understanding and for cultural cooperation: Their development in infancy. In M. Von Cranach, K. Foppa, W. Lepenies, & D. Ploog (Eds.), *Human ethology*. Cambridge: Cambridge University Press.

Trevarthen, C. (1980). Review of: *The making and breaking of affectional bonds* by John Bowlby. *British Journal of Psychiatry, 137,* 390.

Trevarthen, C. (1982). The primary motives for cooperative understanding. In G. Butterworth & P. Light (Eds.), *Studies of the development of understanding*. Chicago: University of Chicago Press.

Trevarthen, C. (1984). Emotions in infancy: Regulators of contact and relationships with persons. In K. R. Scherer & P. Ekman (Eds.), *Approaches to emotion*. Hillsdale, NJ: Erlbaum.

Truffaut, F. (1989). *Autoritratto*. Torino: Einaudi.

Tulving, E. (1972). Episodic and semantic memory. In E. Tulving & W. Donaldson (Eds.), *Organization of memory*. New York: Academic Press.

Tulving, E. (1983). *Elements of episodic memory*. New York: Oxford University Press.

Tulving, E. (1985). How many memory systems are there? *American Psychologist, 40,* 385–398.

Vaillant, G. E. (1977). *Adaptations to life*. Boston: Little, Brown.

Van Den Bergh, O., & Eelen, P. (1984). Unconscious processing and emotions. In M. A. Reda & M. J. Mahoney (Eds.), *Cognitive psychotherapies*. Cambridge, MA: Ballinger.

Varela, F. (1979). *Principles of biological autonomy*. New York: North-Holland.

Varela, F. (1984). The creative cirles: Sketches on the natural history of circularity. In P. Watzlawick (Ed.), *The invented reality.* New York: Norton.

Varela, F. (1987). Laying down a path in walking. In W. J. Thompson (Ed.), *Gaia, a way of knowing.* Great Barrington, MA: Lindisfarne Press.

Weimer, W. B. (1979). *Notes on the methodology of scientific research.* Hillsdale, NJ: Erlbaum.

Weimer, W. B. (1982). Ambiguity and the future of psychology: Meditations leibniziennes. In W. B. Weimer & D. S. Palermo (Eds.), *Cognition and the symbolic processes.* Hillsdale, NJ: Erlbaum.

Weimer, W. B. (1984). Limitations of the dispositional analysis of behavior. In J. R. Royce & L. P. Mos (Eds.), *Annals of theoretical psychology* (Vol. 1). New York: Plenum Press.

Weimer, W. B. (1987). *Rationality in complex orders is never fully explicit nor instantly specifiable.* Unpublished manuscript.

Weissman, M. M., Gammon, G. D., John, K., Merikangas, K. R., Warner, V., Prusoff, B. A., & Sholomskas, D. (1987). Children of depressed parents. *Archives of General Psychiatry, 44,* 847–853.

Weiss, R. S. (1982). Attachment in adult life. In C. M. Parkes & J. Stevenson-Hinde (Eds.), *The place of attachment in human behavior.* London: Tavistock.

Werner, H. (1948). *Comparative psychology of mental development.* New York: International Universities Press.

Werner, H. (1957). The concept of development from a comparative and organismic point of view. In D. E. Harris (Ed.), *The concept of development.* Minneapolis: University of Minnesota Press.

White, P. A. (1980). Limitations on verbal reports of internal events: A refutation of Nisbett and Wilson and of Bem. *Psychological Review, 87,* 105–112.

White, P. A. (1988). Knowing more about what we can tell: "Introspective access" and causal reports accuracy 10 years later. *British Journal of Psychology, 79,* 13–45.

Winograd, T. (1980). What does it mean to understand language? *Cognitive Science, 4,* 209–241.

Winograd, T., & Flores, F. (1986). *Understanding computers and cognition.* Norwood, NJ: Ablex.

Wolf, D. (1982). Understanding others: A longitudinal case study of the concept of independent agency. In G. E. Forman (Ed.), *Action and thought.* New York: Academic Press.

Worden, J. W. (1982). *Grief counseling and grief therapy.* New York: Springer.

Yee, C. M., & Miller, G. A. (1988). Emotional information processing: Modulation of fear in normal and dysthymic subjects. *Journal of Abnormal Psychology, 97,* 54–63. .

Zajonc, R. B. (1984). On primacy of affect. In K. R. Scherer & P. Ekman (Eds.), *Approaches to emotion.* Hillsdale, NJ: Erlbaum.

Zajonc, R. B., & Markus, H. (1984). Affect and cognition: The hard interface. In C. E. Izard, J. Kagan, & R. B. Zajonc (Eds.), *Emotions, cognition and behavior.* Cambridge: Cambridge University Press.

Zambrano, M. (1988). *Persona y democracia* (pp. 62–63). Barcelona: Anthropos. (Original work published 1958)

Zeleny, M. (Ed.). (1981). *Autopoiesis: A theory of living organization.* New York: North-Holland.

Zisook, S. (Ed.). (1988). Emotional information processing: Modulation of fear in normal and dystymic subjects. *Journal of Abnormal Psychology, 97,* 54–63.

Zubin, J., Steinhauer, S. R., Day, R., & van Kammen, D. P. (1985). Schizophrenia at the crossroads: A blueprint for the 1980s. In M. Alpert (Ed.), *Controversies in schizophrenia.* New York: Guilford Press.

Index